What Do I
Do While **You're**
Pregnant?

Kenny Bodanis

Library and Archives Canada Cataloguing in Publication

Bodanis, Kenny, 1971-, author
      What do I do while you're pregnant? / Kenny Bodanis.
Previous title: Men get pregnant, too.
Issued in print and electronic formats.
ISBN   978-0-9936140-2-6   (paperback).--ISBN   978-0-9936140-3-3 (pdf)

            1. Bodanis, Kenny, 1971-.   2. Pregnancy--Popular works.
3. Pregnancy--Humor.   4. Pregnant women--Relations with men--
Popular works. 5. Men--Psychology--Popular works. 6. Fathers--
Psychology--Popular Works.   I. Bodanis, Kenny, 1971- . Men get
pregnant, too. II. Title.
RG525.B632 2015   618.2'4   C2015-905647-0

                                                  C2015-905648-9

Printed in Canada & the United States of America.
© 2015 Kenny Bodanis

Cover Layout & Design: Antony Vannapho
Interior design: Christine Keleny, ckbookspublishing.com

For Dale:

My love through all of life's labors.

Why write this book?

"Men don't contribute much to relationships, and women no longer need them to be the breadwinners. Then, they blame feminism for their failure to evolve. They need to stop whining like a bunch of sissies and be the man a woman would want to be with. They're hard to find in this new world because men refuse to adapt."

Letter from "Angie" to the *Chicago Sun-Times*. February 3rd, 2011

Table of Contents

About This Book

I wrote this book to create my own little empathetic friend with whom I could cuddle and to whom I could complain throughout my wife's pregnancy. Naturally, my hopes for this little collection of pages was that it would also become a beacon of understanding not only for fathers-to-be feeling out of place—with only potato chips to grow *their* bellies during their wives' pregnancies—but also as a gentle nudge for expectant mothers whose husbands may not have yet found their strongest voice during the 40 weeks of gestation. I wanted to encourage those men to express themselves and to be receptive about their *own* emotional and physical changes during this period.

Hindsight is 20/20, they say. Never more so than when a Parenting Blogger gets the chance to insert some fatherly wisdom into a book that speaks of his journey as a parent-to-be. I have two children now and have used blogging as one outlet through which I could develop my voice.

Some of these 'I'm a Dad, now, so I've learned a bunch of stuff' epiphanies are included in this book as inserts entitled: "Back From the Future – From Blog to Book."

A few of these bits of wisdom are drawn from my MenGetPregnantToo.com blog posts. Others are drawn from my day-to-day experiences as a father who just can't *wait* for the next tantrum or the next meatloaf rejection due to the flecks of green hidden within it or the next moment of hurtful disobedience from someone who still sleeps with a stuffed duck.

Enjoy this book, and good luck with all that other stuff.

Introduction

It's time. Time for a frank conversation about what women perceive as one of men's shortcomings but what men know is an alternate truth we're too chicken to talk about. That truth is this: becoming a parent for the first time is daunting and scary for men, too.

This is not in the biological sense, but emotionally and psychologically we feel stress, nervousness, anxiety, sadness (yes, even post-partum depression), euphoria and, at times, outright fear at the prospect of becoming a new parent.

The conundrum we face is: progressive values scold men for not being in touch with their "Female Brain." Meanwhile, the *iDADs* (Dads with Emotional Intelligence) are growing in number and facing a different reality. We are part of a change in gender roles; a groundswell of fathers who are adapting happily to a shift in the family dynamic that understands that domestic chores and hands-on parenting need not be restricted to a particular sex.

However, this dynamic is still far from being tacitly accepted as a workable model. At dinner parties, at cafe gatherings, at Mom and Tot groups, as well as at play-dates with friends, the following conversation is frequently repeated:

The Pregnant Mother: "Sometimes I'm just so tired; I feel nauseous all the time, my appetite comes and goes and I feel completely unattractive. Men are so lucky, once the sex is done, for them it's nine months of television and leisure time until the baby's born and then more of the same while my breasts become udders."

Most iDADs I know are experiencing a quiet firestorm of angst. They are blindly playing 'best-guess.' They are trying to take over household chores without getting in the way. They are also searching for the right combinations of teas, foot massages, backrubs and over-the-counter painkillers that will make their pregnant wives comfortable, confident and stress-free. They are aware that helping their wives mentally and physically relax is in the best interest of the mother, the fetus and themselves.

But beneath this facade is a man struggling to deal with feelings he may have never experienced and questions for which he desperately wants answers:

- Am I allowed to feel depressed and nervous, too?
- I know my wife is uncomfortable, but what more can I do?
- Can I be the type of father my baby deserves?

The iDAD's voice is not always welcome within round-table discussions during his wife's pregnancy. A father-to-be's admission that he has had trouble sleeping due to nerves related to impending parenthood usually yields the following response:

-"Phullease! You're not the one who has to squeeze something the size of a watermelon out of a hole the size of a ping pong ball."

True.

How do you compete with that? It's as though the championship game is being played and you're not even allowed on the field with the team. This is especially true when your biological shortcoming is hoisted onto the table: We have never, nor will we ever be able to, become pregnant.

But here is the iDAD's truth: We do as much as we can.

And, at the end of the day, we are also tired; we are also scared the baby may not be healthy and that the mother may not be happy. We are scared by the knowledge that we will share 50 percent of the responsibility of this child's upbringing for the rest of our lives. We want our children to have friends and to be generous with others and to be able to say "I love you" and do well in school. We want all that while also still wanting them to look forward to coming home for dinner with their parents. All of these things are like a ball of rubber bands sitting in our gut. Socially, most male relationships with their peers have not yet evolved to the point where they can cry to their male friends about their worries. It's just not done. Yes, it's unfortunate, and no doubt it will change in a generation or two. But, for now, it's a duality that exists: The doubts and feelings are there, but the opportunities to express them and the existence of support networks, are scarce.

The irony is this: The iDAD's football buddy is down the street, feeling exactly the same range of anxious emotions. Like other iDADs, he is also reluctant to burden his pregnant wife with his concerns.

While there is a "Dear Abby," there has yet to be a "Dear Chuck."

So, no, we have no uterus. So, yes, we can still keep down leftover pizza for breakfast during the first trimester. But, stress headaches? You bet. Phantom symptoms? Yep.

The question I asked most during those nine months was, how do I handle it all?

What Do I Do While You're Pregnant?

CHAPTER 1
Ready To Be a Parent

- PET PEEVE OF THE iDAD -

Being called nothing more than a sperm donor.

I was first married at 24 years old; it lasted less than four years. Thankfully, we did not have children together— although discussions had begun. We had become 'one of those': an unhappily married couple still entertaining thoughts of having a baby. I know now the reason we talked about kids was the same reason we married: It was simply what we felt was expected of us. Before we married, we were together for nearly two years and eager to be accepted as adults. People started to ask: "So, is this the one?" I didn't want to admit I wasn't sure; I felt that wasn't the answer people wanted to hear. I had been accepted into a family that was comfortable, warm and loving. Although my girlfriend and I seemed to bicker and maintain a constant level of tension in our relationship, there were reassurances that this was a normal side-effect of being young, as well as being full-time students. We were convinced things would settle down in time.

So...onward with the wedding plans.

Two years into the marriage, things were still not going well. But the next logical question was already being fired at us from all directions:

-"So when will we see a little grandchild at the Christmas table?"

You certainly don't have the strength of character at 24 years old to look your in-laws in the eye and tell them you have been fighting a lot and that you're not sure things are going to work out, and the baby-making will have to wait until after the marriage counseling. Especially when these in-laws, by-and-large, paid five figures for a wedding ceremony and reception for 130 guests.

Instead, you go home and talk about it.

You repeat the lines you've heard as bits of wisdom after each argument you've had as a married couple:

- "Everyone says the first year can be tough, and it will only get better after that."

- "It's normal to still be adjusting to married life; things will be easier once we've settled down."

Fortunately, things got bad enough soon enough that we separated before making a run at parenthood. Only now do I know what a blessing that decision was.

Having been a child growing up in a house with a fair amount of arguing taking place on the other side of my bedroom wall, I knew my child deserved more than to be born to parents who weren't getting along even *before* they were married.

§

Years later I remarried. *This* felt right. It felt *easy.* Ironically, when we got married, neither of us was sure we would ever want children. Once again, about 18 months passed and the families started asking questions, this time a little more earnestly. I was pushing 30 and my wife was six years my senior:

- "Where's the baby?"

My wife couldn't turn down a glass of wine or have an

afternoon nap on a Sunday without our families launching an investigation worthy of the FBI into whether this outrageous behavior may be due to her new condition. And, much like J. Edgar Hoover, my family did not worry about invasion of privacy: "Is she pregnant?!" they would demand.

A word to members of our parents' generation who may be overcome by wishful thinking related to grandchildren: If your children have not told you they are expecting a baby, chances are they are not expecting a baby. If they *are* expecting a baby and have not told you about it, it is because THEY DON'T WANT YOU TO KNOW. Why? It could be any one of several reasons. Perhaps they want to evaluate for themselves how they feel about their new baby. Maybe they're worried about your re-action: Will you be overbearing? Disappointed? Will you insist on moving into their home along with a never-ending supply of lasagna? Will you call them three times a day to find out whether the fetus has kicked?

The reasons may be more serious, such as a medical condi-tion that threatens the mother or the baby; one that affects the couple's decision on whether to go through with the pregnancy (more on that point later in the book).

In our case, our reaction to their questions about pregnancy was—in their eyes—the worst news possible. If you ever want to see a look of disappointment on your parents' faces, tell them you're not sure if you *ever* want to have children. Ouch.

But my wife and I were older and more able to deal with stares, 'tsk-tsks,' and the truth that my family tree may grow no more branches once my siblings and I were gone (my siblings were about as far from being parents as Napoleon and Josephine were from reconciliation).

My wife and I were textbook 'D.I.N.K.s' (Double-Income-No-Kids): work, late movies, late dinners, a bottle of wine or two and general childless debauchery. The thought of us being co-pilots of a mini-van made our skin crawl. We just looked at those parents driving an hour to and from work, trying to park their minivans and SUVs in tiny downtown spots, unable to go for a walk in the woods because it interferes with naptime. THAT was no kind of life.

But then a few months into our marriage, a strange thing happened: when we were around children—whether they were infants, toddlers or teens—we felt something stir. When we stared at kids, our faces were overcome by 'the look'—our heads tilted, our eyes softened and the edges of our mouths curved upwards slightly. Suddenly we began to see the fulfilling side of giving birth to, and nourishing, and raising, and sharing one's life with these little humans.

And the discussions began.

§

We shared the same fears vis-à-vis parenthood.

We both had the unfortunate privilege of working for local media outlets. Because good news doesn't sell, we saw, on a daily basis, the worst of what the world offered the 21st century child: drugs, violence, drop-outs, gangs, violent movies and video games, junk food, kidnappers, pedophiles, reckless drivers, fires and floods. And that was just within the broadcast's first fifteen minutes.

How could two individuals compete with the onslaught that would await our child once he or she walked out the front door? The burden of being responsible for the care, safety, self-esteem and development of a human being—from scratch!—made us very nervous.

So we talked. We pro'd and con'd. We discussed and analyzed. Could we afford it? How much money *makes* it affordable? Were we ready to give up our lifestyle? There would be no such thing as 'sleeping in' for the next decade or so—and I *loved* to sleep in (I still do, I just can't anymore, so I made adjustments. It's amazing how functional one can be while still maintaining a low-level, fatigue-induced fog. You can all thank me later for not becoming a surgeon; the lawsuits would have bankrupted me for sure). Are we ready to be devoted to another human being for every minute of every day, whether they were at home or at a friend's house, whether they were healthy or sick, happy or sad, failing or succeeding?

We always came to the same conclusions: We felt being *aware* of all these trappings gave us the necessary framework to begin *considering* parenthood and that parenthood was something we now both wanted—something we both *needed.* The biological tickle was undeniable.

Were we ready? Who knows? What's "ready" anyway? The truth is this: Readiness reveals itself when you're alone at night with your thoughts. Only *you* know what is going through your mind when you consider life as a parent. The real challenge—what requires strength and honesty—is not trying to convince yourself or your spouse of anything different during waking hours.

Personally, these things *did* keep me awake at night. Could I be the type of father a child deserved to have? There was a litany of stories from armchair fathers whose job it was simply to have an office job: to work 9 to 5, deposit the paycheck and to then take care of his second set of obligations, which consisted of household manual labor. Sure, they took out the garbage, they trimmed the hedges and they built decks. Other than that, Dad was not to be disturbed, not to be pulled out of the armchair—especially when the game was on.

How could I teach my son that girls, and eventually women, should be treated with care and respect? How could I convince him that he, too, is deserving of that same care and respect?

How could I teach my daughter to believe in herself, to rely on her confidence and her abilities and to work at developing whatever stokes her passion? How do you teach someone to love *themselves* as much as those people who are important to them?

I know boys—I was one. Sex is a powerful driving force. I broke into a cold sweat when I thought of my teenage son fathering a child. And how could I teach my daughter that teenage boys *do* tend to think of only one thing: sex? How would I teach her that, at fifteen, when he says "I love you," he does not always mean he loves you? Even when it is sincere, his love is young love and will not last forever, and the consequences of believing it will be disastrous. I remember my parents warning me of those things, and I remember believing with every fiber of my being that they were wrong. I met the woman of my dreams at least four times before I turned 15. Fortunately, I was too shy, or perhaps just shy enough, not to do anything stupid.

I smoked tobacco. I smoked pot. I smoked hash. I ate magic mushrooms and I drank—sometimes to excess. I drove while under the influences of all of the above. I narrowly escaped disaster more times than I can count—despite my mother believing she could "always tell when I was lying." How could I possibly keep my kid safe? What special skill-set did I have that would keep my child from making that *one* mistake they would regret for the rest of their lives?

I did horribly in school. I never listened. I was a smart-ass and was nearly expelled for poor grades in nearly every single semester of high school. Why would I do homework when I could watch "Happy Days" and "Taxi" while eating a bowl of peanut butter with a spoon? I was convinced I was going to win an Oscar by age 25—what does an actor need with Physics, Chemistry, Math and English? Will my child be the smart-ass who will defend himself with: "*You* only have a High School education, and you turned out all right."? How would I impart a philosophy I believe in without turning them off and pushing them to rebellion by sounding too preachy and hypocritical?

All this was going through my head before I donated a single sperm. Who knew a man could complicate sex so much?

I was told repeatedly by friends and colleagues, the fact that I was questioning myself in the first place meant I was headed in the right direction. I looked around and saw there are nearly seven billion people on the planet, many of whom managed to raise competent children, and some of whom turned parenting into an unmitigated disaster.

But at night, when my wife and I were alone with our own thoughts, we both thought the same thing. My wife and I finally acknowledged we no longer could imagine a life without children.

It was time to make a baby.

˙ SELF-REFLECTION TIP FOR THE iDAD ˙

Don't deny what your inner voice knows to be true.

BACK FROM THE FUTURE

From Blog to Book

Inspired by the MenGetPregnantToo.com Post:
That Baby-Hater is Dancing With My Baby!
Published: November 1, 2012.

11

There are many people who make a *choice* not to have children. One of them is my sister's best friend, Annie Thomas. Although Annie and I have known each other for more than thirty years, we were never close enough to discuss the fact she and her husband of more than a decade have no children. That question is none of anybody's business. But as I mentioned in a post I wrote in the week following a conversation with Annie at my sister's wedding, it's a question parents *always* want to ask childless couples. It was also a question Annie had been dogged with for more than a decade: At my sister's wedding on Sunday I was chatting with one of her closest friends. She asked if I had read her article published on TheScrib.com: "Confessions of a Baby Hater."

Annie is my age and has also been married for 10 years. She has about fourteen dogs (OK, she has two or three dogs. But to those of us with *no* canine family members, more than one dog equates to exponentially excessive quantities of hair, drool and nasty breath) but no children.

I always wondered why. Now, after reading her post, I know why: She never *wanted* them.

Imagine!

When I'm with D.I.N.K.s, (Double-Income-No-Kids) I become sensitive about their space and about how my kids may be infringing upon it (something I wish more dog owners would do). If they wanted to have kids, but were unable to, I don't want my children to trigger unhappy memories. If they, like

Annie and her husband, made a *choice* to remain childless, it may be because they would rather *not* have little monkeys like mine climbing into their laps, asking for rides on their feet or sharing their French fries. We parents *always* wonder why D.I.N.K.s don't have children. It's really none of our business. But as Annie points out in her post, that doesn't stop people:

"When you're single everyone asks you when you are going to get married (for which the appropriate answer is: when I find a boyfriend, dickwad) and when you are married everyone asks you when you are going to have children. My long standing answer was always "I don't believe in those things." Most people don't know what to do with that answer and generally shut their pie holes thereafter on the subject."

I think, secretly, parents are infinitely curious about child-less couples. Partly because there are (hopefully a minority) of mommies and daddies who would have made different choices, but felt trapped. As the "Baby-Hater" points out, the statistics don't support our version of 'happily ever-after':

"Entering full-blown adulthood, it started to become evident that most people were following some kind of a "life" roadmap. Get married by 25, buy a house at 27, have the first of 2.3 children shortly thereafter. 50 percent to get divorced at 35."

13

Having a failed marriage does not mean one wishes they never had children. However, I've heard many parents who have shared custody of their sons and daughters and treat their weekend with the kids as an inconvenience.

My point is this: There is no right or wrong when it comes to choosing whether to have children. There are plenty of parents who should never have had children—just ask their kids. There are also bushels of D.I.N.K.s whose tenderness, selflessness, empathy and maturity would make them natural mothers and fathers. The fact that they choose *not* to have offspring is no shame; those people improve the planet simply by being decent human beings.

So being with my children at my sister's wedding I was mindful of Annie—the Baby-Hating blog-writer—and her husband. I was careful to prevent them from experiencing the claustrophobia of having my offspring climb on their laps and stand on their shoes. I felt protective of their privacy. They didn't want children. They *certainly* didn't want mine.

My perspective changed once Annie and my 5-year-old daughter hit the dance floor.

The two of them developed instant chemistry as they let their "Backbone Slide," and they "Ice-Ice Baby" 'ed. My daughter romped as Annie stomped. They grabbed hands and made each other nauseous as they twirled around the center of the bar. It was clear the two ladies—32 years apart in age—shared a kinship. They are both confident people, sure about their choices, and they both make no apologies for non-conformity.

Annie doesn't hate kids. She hates *annoying* kids. On that

point, she and I agree, especially since chronic annoyingness in children is usually born of similar traits in their parents. Annie also hates being frowned upon for sculpting a lifestyle which includes adult time, HBO at 8 p.m. and dependants who only need to be fed, walked, brushed and to have their poop fall onto a sidewalk instead of into a diaper.

CHAPTER 2
When Sex Becomes Homework

· PET PEEVE OF THE iDAD ·

Assuming men can never have enough sex.

S o there we go! Yes sir, baby-makin' time! I remember, as an adolescent, looking at married couples and thinking to myself: "Wow, they get to have sex whenever they want. Every day. Twice a day. He gets to look at her boobs and touch them, and she *lets* him."

Yadda, yadda.

Sex can be wonderful, mind-blowing, passionate, hot, caring and blissful. It can also be homework. Yes, even for men.

Stereotypical, degrading myth: "Men can get an erection when the wind blows or when the Super Bowl pre-game show begins."

At 17 years old? Yes. Now add a decade or two, a full time job, taxes, garbage day, cooking and cleaning, and a deadline for sexual performance. Suddenly...Not so much.

The very first time we made love for the Purpose of Reproduction (how's *that* for sexy talk?), I felt a deep emotional reaction. Pardon the Harlequin metaphor, but we *did* look into each other's eyes and recognize that something more important than us was taking place. There was an extra layer added to our lifelong bond that came from knowing we were entering a different and more complex relationship. We were working towards forever being someone's mother and father. I felt a deeper sense of belonging and purpose than I had ever thought possible.

Procreative rolls-in-the-hay for the first month or so were

often followed by playful discussions of various mom and dad scenarios we would face in the coming years:

- "Can you imagine someone calling you 'Mummy'?"

- "Can you believe we'll be helping our own kid with their homework?"

- "I can't wait to rub little feet while we read the baby a bedtime story."

Occasionally anxiety crept in:

- "Do you think we're doing the right thing?"

I still laugh at that now, because I would often bravely reassure my wife by boasting that we cannot second-guess ourselves; as long as we know this is something we both want, we need to exude positive energy and have faith.

Oh, brave fool.

Inside, I was Woody Allen meets SpongeBob SquarePants: a nervous wreck.

Eventually, a month turned into two, then three, then four. Should it be taking this long?

As a child growing up, our family spoke openly about sexuality. My mother was a nurse; the human body, and all of its functions, were nothing to be ashamed of. A penis was a penis not a "member" or a "Johnson." A vagina was a vagina. Sex was sex. I was an early reader, and as soon as I could understand written language, I remember being handed two books: "Where Did I Come From?" and "What's Happening to Me?" The latter explained—nude photos included—the various stages of puberty; the former—though only cartoon portraits this time—detailed intercourse, ejaculation and pregnancy. I was suffi-ciently terrified of the prospect of becoming a teenage dad that I didn't lose my virginity until I was almost nineteen.

Now, as an adult, I was having almost tiresome amounts of sex *solely* for the purpose of procreation, and it wasn't working. Oh, the irony. I was sure the only explanation for this lack of procreation must be some form of physical malfunction. Bless the era of self-help literature. It was time to do some research.

All the expert opinions I read said it can *easily* take six months to conceive your first child. Apparently subsequent babies come more easily; one of the explanations being the woman's body is more prepared for pregnancy the second time, having been through it once before. *I* believe the reason lies more with nature giving you more time before the first one in order to really give you a chance to think about it and to possibly back out of this lifelong obligation. After this waiting period, should you choose to ignore the warnings from friends about sleepless nights and mysterious infant behavior, nature throws you into the parental lion's den: You apparently still want it badly enough; go ahead and have as many as you want, we'll make it easier for any subsequent children.

After playing amateur conception sleuth for a week or so after a prolonged period of ineffective sex, we realized the solution was obvious: more sex. This was the teenager's dream mutated into something completely different.

Was it only 20 years ago I was resenting being a full-time student, largely because I couldn't stand the homework, and I envied married people because they got to have sex whenever they wanted? Well, guess what? I was getting the best of both worlds now.

Mathematics dictated, if we made love every second day

for a month, one of tens of millions of sperm would eventually have no choice but to meet an egg. If we did it too often—daily, for instance—my sperm count would not have a chance to increase between ejaculations. If it was done too seldom—every third or fourth day, for instance—we might miss the ovulation window. Charming. Statistics motivated and reassured us; even if it's on holiday schedule, the bus will arrive eventually, your job is just to keep showing up at the stop—every second day—until it does.

Women often explain that after a full day of work, be it domestic or corporate, the last thing they want to do is use what little energy they have left to please their husbands, who seem to have limitless interest in sex.

Well, guess what? Men get tired, too.

My job had me waking up at 3:15 in the morning. I was the producer of a full-service morning show: news, weather, traffic, sports and daily doses of the latest medical information. The majority of staff members working with me behind the scenes were women of child-bearing age. It seemed there wasn't a three-month period that passed without someone either announcing their pregnancy or going on maternity leave. I worked at a baby factory, yet *my* machinery was failing.

One of the few advantages to completing most of my workday before sunrise was I was often able to be home by noon. However, much like a shift worker, my body's rhythms had gone haywire. My energy peaked at five in the morning. It was at that period of my day I always had lofty ideas about going on a long afternoon walk with my wife, making inspirational and inventive love all afternoon, and cooking a romantic dinner.

But after a 10 a.m. breakfast in the corporate cafeteria, I always started to crash. By the time I came home, I was exhausted. I was starving for what seemed to be my fourteenth meal of the day (ideally potato chips or breakfast cereal), and I yearned for a long afternoon nap.

-"Today's *'a day'*." My wife would say to remind me that 48 hours had passed since we last had sex.

OK, I would say. I'll just close my eyes for an hour, and I'll be fine. We can roll in the hay later this afternoon.

One hour would turn into two – bless her; she would let me sleep.

I always woke up feeling like I was battling a college hangover; I needed two aspirin, more food and more sleep. Nothing makes a man feel less attractive than having bed-head and morning breath in the middle of the afternoon. Try initiating sex when you feel like you've just arrived home after four connecting flights from Southeast Asia. Men don't talk about this, but from time to time we also need to feel attractive to get turned on. Aside from my own feelings, I'm sure in that condition I presented a heavenly vision for my wife. I'll bet she couldn't control herself and she just *had* to have me. But if I didn't also initiate sex occasionally, we might be D.I.N.K.s forever.

Of course, the definition of 'initiate' changes when sex is on the calendar more frequently than it is on your mind. It becomes more acknowledgement and capitulation than desire and lust.

Believe it or not, emotional involvement when making love does make men better lovers. If I don't feel attractive, confident and sexy before jumping into the sack, there are consequences: shorter duration, temporary erectile dysfunction and becoming somewhat robotic are just a few of them. And, yes, it bothers me because, yes, I care. It's not all about the orgasm for men, either. I knew I wasn't the only one being worn down by repetition. Knowing my wife would probably rather be gardening than making love made me feel very sheepish and guilty before, during and after the act. Of course, she was marvelously supportive and realistic. She knew to appeal to the statistical side of my brain:

-"Look, when you're having sex fifteen times a month, I don't expect you to be Superman. Believe me, I have to force myself sometimes, too."

That always comforted me, except maybe for that last part.

Ask men how often they talk to their buddies about sporadic, fatigue-and-stress-induced erectile dysfunction. Never. Unless you happen to be blessed with a friend who has been like a brother since the seventh grade. Rob was the one person I knew who both had testicles and could stand to hear and speak the truth. A couple of months into the 'Let's Make a Baby' tour, I asked Rob what it was like when he and his wife were trying for their first:

-"Oh, it can be horrible; like homework. You just have to hunker down, commit, run upstairs to the bedroom for as long as it takes to get the job done and hope to hell it took."

I felt like a woman in a shampoo commercial: A soft wind blew through my hair, music played and flowers bloomed. My sexual dysfunction wasn't so much a dysfunction as it was a reality which existed for anyone with a full time job (be it domestic or corporate) and was having difficulty procreating. I

23

wasn't alone. My feelings had been validated by another healthy male. I was a new man—until my alarm went off the next morning at 3:15.

§

Human beings are funny. We can go to a Black Tie Event and be told by the Queen of England and her entire court we look dashingly handsome in our tuxedo, but if later in the evening a child points out a pimple on our forehead, what Elizabeth II said doesn't mean squat; we tend to lend more weight to something negative than something positive.

All it took was one more session of overly-practical, 100-meter dash love-making to give my self-esteem a good kick in the pants. After several weeks of diligent, scheduled, sex-with-a-purpose, it was a shame the time my wife spent reassuring me wasn't being applied toward a psychiatry degree she could use later on; if we never ended up having kids, at least being married to a doctor would probably pay for a top-of-the-line home theater.

Yes, men are vain; but to what extent we keep hidden. The less success I was having in the sack, the more time I would spend in front of the mirror noticing the appearances of Love Handles (an ironic name for a new body part, considering the circumstances), hairs where there were none before, and, yes, wrinkles. Perhaps I was infertile due to some bizarre rapid aging syndrome. I was Dorian Gray *without* the portrait in the attic or viable sperm.

Self-esteem is like a set of Dominoes, whether you're full of testosterone, estrogen, or something else entirely, once you begin to doubt yourself, there is an exponential cascading effect.

I prepared myself for the truth that our having children maybe just wasn't meant to be.

In the meantime, the relatives kept hammering away:

- "So, when will we see grandchildren?"
- "So, when will we see some nieces or nephews?"
- "So, when will we see some cousins?"

We didn't dare be truthful. If I had to choose between telling our parents we might be infertile or placating them with excuses until death do us part, the latter was the easy winner.

Occasionally I did lose my cool. Although my issuing a firm reminder that they would be the first to know if we were expecting usually worked (yes, I said the same thing to no matter whom I was talking: that they would *all* be the first to know), I would find myself blowing up from time to time:

-"What if we told you we couldn't have kids?!"

Silence. That got 'em.

They would invariably step back and ask if that were true; the same answer would follow:

-"You'll know when we know." Now, back off! I have to go have sex.

They would keep their inquisitive distance for another six weeks. But sometimes my own voice would resonate within me, and on the way home we would ask ourselves that same question:

-"What if we can't have kids?"

Six months had come and gone. It was time to visit the fertility clinic.

· ROMANCE TIP FOR THE iDAD ·

Especially when trying every second day for months to make a baby,
surprise your wife once a week with anything that
will break up the routine.

CHAPTER 3:

Where the Orgasm Meets the Receptionist

My wife and I didn't seem to be able to conceive a child. It was time to discover whether, biologically speaking, it was either her fault or mine or both. It was time for tests.

Step one was to report to the hospital's fertility clinic. We were amazed to find the waiting room was standing room only. The room was a cross-section of our planet's human population: a melting pot of couples of different races, ages and religious beliefs; couples composed of a mom and a dad or two moms or two dads, all sitting in silence watching CNN on the television suspended from the ceiling or reading *MacLean's* magazine or sipping coffee dispensed from an unattractive square brown machine in the corner. No couples were talking; neither to each other, nor to anyone else.

There are topics that, culturally, we have all been taught are nobody else's business. Among them are our income, how much debt we have accrued, how often we fight or have sex, and information about a member of the family who has an illness. Infertility is another.

What a shame.

The anguish for couples struggling to get pregnant could be lessened tenfold if we felt comfortable sharing it with family and friends. I think this is even truer of being able to share it with a stranger sitting next to you at the fertility clinic. We each spent months secretly worrying about the family we may never have, only to walk into a room filled with human beings who have been meeting with experts for months, hoping to find a solution to a similar problem. Sitting in that room was like being in a prison and not asking your cellmate what he's in for.

One reason we keep to ourselves is the fear of becoming a sideshow for the curious. There is a difference between being supportive and being nosey.

A difference between—

- "I'm sorry to hear that. How are you feeling? Let me know if there is anything I can do, and please feel free to talk about it if you need to share."

And—

- "So?"

- "Any news?"

- "What's the next step?

- "So, any more news?"

- "My cousin had the same thing."

And the dreaded—

- "I hope you don't mind, but I mentioned your problem to a friend of mine whose sister had the same problem. They ended up adopting two beautiful Chinese boys."

They never tell you about the $25,000 price tag for the adoption, or the tens-of-thousands of dollars spent on fertility treatments, or the devastation of preparing a baby-room only to have the adoption fall through at the last minute. Nor are they able to discuss and comfort you with the real crisis: The emotional strain of dealing with—and accepting—the fact that you seem biologically incapable of creating life.

Yet, here we were, sitting in silence next to our stressed, childless peers.

We met with a doctor who asked us general questions about our health. He asked how often and with what frequency we had sex, as well as a battery of other routine questions.

My wife's gynecologist had her on Clomid—the trade name of Clomiphene, a common fertility drug for women taken in pill form. According to the reproductive specialist counseling us at the clinic—who was also an OBGYN—my wife had been taking the drug for too long and had not undergone the proper tests before being prescribed the drug in the first place. Thank you very much, Dr. Months-of-Our-Lives-Wasted. We immediately asked the doctor in front of us if he was taking on new patients. Yes, he said, as long as we were patients of the fertility clinic he could see my wife for regular examinations, as well.

He answered all of our questions with the most sympathetic tone I'd ever heard in a doctor's office. He seemed to anticipate our every concern and allay most of our fears. It was clear that we were one of thousands of patients coming to him with what are—at least at this stage—routine problems. So routine, nobody talks about them.

He did say we may have a long road ahead of us. Should the first few routine procedures not bear fruit, the wait could be long and the cost could be high. But he encouraged us to relax and not put the cart before the horse.

After external exams revealed nothing out of the ordinary, we were both scheduled for blood and urine tests. My wife was scheduled for a hysterosalpingogram or HSG. This is a procedure during which fluid is injected past the opening of the cervix and an x-ray examines more closely the uterus and fallopian tubes. This has the advantage of being able to check for blockages or abnormalities that may impede the egg from making the journey from the ovary to the uterus. My wife was warned this procedure involved a certain level of discomfort and possibly even pain. She was told it would be similar to an intense period cramp. Friends of hers, who had had the test done before, warned her that comparing this to a period cramp was like comparing Goliath to David. Great.

I was scheduled to return to give a sperm sample; the procedure being locking myself in a room and masturbating into a cup. Ma'am, you'll undergo a painful medical procedure; sir, you orgasm into this Petri dish. She: 1, Me: 0.

According to my wife, the HSG procedure was as described by the physician, but the pain did not quite live up to the popular hysteria. It was three minutes of severe period cramps while the x-rays were taken. She admitted it was not at all comfortable, but it was definitely not the torture some of her peers had described. I'm sure, as with all things (conception included), the experience is unique to each person.

Next, it was my turn. I reported to a 'private' clinic, which was three thousand square feet of open office space with two walls of floor-to-ceiling windows, facing one of the city's busiest streets, and my mother worked as a nurse in the hospital across the street. Private clinic, indeed. Were my mother's hospital windows facing my clinic windows? I could imagine her shouting across the boulevard through the screen: "Kenny! What are you doing in a private lab?! WHAT!? I CAN'T HEAR

YOU WITH ALL THIS TRAFFIC! HANG ON! I'LL COME OVER THERE!"

Lining the walls of the clinic's foyer were office chairs around a large rug that served as a waiting area. There were magazine racks full of short-term literature to entertain patients (clients?), significant others, or some very loyal friends along for moral support while the donors...donated.

On the opposite side of the waiting room was a glass partition behind which was *The Lab*. I had a clear view of technicians in white coats scurrying about, ironically much like the sperm in Woody Allen's *Everything You Always Wanted to Know About Sex *But Were Afraid to Ask*. They shuffled Petri dishes, beakers and syringes like cards in a casino. That morning's crop of sperm-donors had long since gone home and was now waiting by their phones for results. Those results would be positive or negative or benign or malignant. These backstage Oompa Loompas in lab coats were handing out destinies one phone call at a time.

I have never felt so grateful for having the reason for my appointment written on a prescription pad so it did not have to be spoken aloud. I handed the script to the receptionist, who, for some reason, was also wearing a lab coat. (Why do medical receptionists also behave as though they're MDs?) She offered no greeting; no 'Hello,' no 'How are you today, sir?' no sympathy at all for the future donor standing before her. Like a car being registered, my personal information was entered into her computer. I was now a client on file:

Client 12345: Kenny Bodanis Sperm Donation
Possibly Infertile

Definitely Nervous.

I signed. I paid. I was handed a cup large enough to hold a stack of a dozen-or-so quarters. I tried to keep my expression neutral as the blood pooled in my face. Given the fact that I could hear my heartbeat pulsating in my ears, I was fairly certain I was blushing. When you're about to have sex with your wife, the blood rushes to your penis; when you're about to donate sperm in a lab, it rushes to your cheeks—how unfair. There was nothing to do about it except explain that my rosacea prescription was in my other coat pocket.

I asked Nurse Ratched for the location of *the room*. She said there was a washroom directly across from the reception area.

A bathroom. *A bathroom?* Off the *reception area?* No bed, no adult magazines, no soft music, no movies, no candle light, no motivational speaker on staff, no words of encouragement at all; just a washroom directly off a waiting room, next to a processing lab. Sexy.

I tried to get my wife's attention, trying to campaign for some sympathy for the sad clown who was headed to the bathroom to masturbate into a plastic change cup. She nodded and smiled at me with the same supportive look my buddy gave me when my ear was pierced in high school ("Thumbs up! It'll look awesome! So what if it never heals?"). She had already made herself comfortable with the latest edition of *People* magazine.

§

All men masturbate. All of us. Regularly. Ask your man if

he masturbates and there is a better than average chance he will dance around the answer, change the topic or outright lie. The answer is yes. If he says he has, but not in a long while, he's lying. Male masturbation is a confusing issue between men and women. For some reason, everyone feels uncomfortable talking about it, the same way people get sheepish when saying the word 'vagina.' They always downgrade to a secretive whisper, as though masturbation and vaginas have been illegally imported. Men are afraid to admit to their girlfriends and wives that they masturbate because they are worried it will be perceived as cheating.

- "Aren't I enough for you?" they say. Or—
- "Why do you have to masturbate?"

And the inevitable (and dreaded)—

- "Do you think of *me* when you masturbate?"

Sit down and make yourself comfortable; here is the truth about male masturbation:

We do it because we can. We do it because there is a penis hanging between our legs, and when we take two or five or ten minutes to massage it in a certain way, it feels quite good. It is like mountain climbing—we do it because it's there. But, unlike a mountain, masturbation carries with it next to no risk of injury or death, and we don't need a helmet to do it. I think the confusion is created because men have not succeeded in explaining to women that masturbation has nothing to do with feelings. Not our feeling towards ourselves, not our feelings towards our wives, not our feelings towards our families. Masturbation has as much to do with how much we love our refrigerators as it does with how much we love our lovers. There is absolutely no correlation.

It also has nothing to do with how much sex we are having with another human being. It's true. Believe it or not. You could be engaging in physical love-making with your man daily, twice-daily or (phew!) even more often than that, and he would still find the time to masturbate. And when he says he loves you more than life itself and can't wait to spend the next sixty years with you in wedded bliss, he is telling the truth. Loving the act of pleasuring himself and loving you are completely unrelated. There. Have dinner and discuss, then leave it alone and never mention it again.

Clinical sperm donation, on the other hand, is a different story. There is definitely not the same motivation to donate sperm in a lab as there is to masturbate at home, despite the orgasm.

§

The washroom was like many other public washrooms: big enough for a wheelchair; a low sink with oversized handles; support bars on the wall. It was tiled in that mild, clinically inoffensive green normally reserved for public hospitals, private clinics and aliens on "Star Trek". They say that color is supposed to relax you. Wine is relaxing. *On Golden Pond* is relaxing. This color made me wonder if it was chosen due to its effectiveness at hiding mold.

I examined myself in the mirror for no reason other than to stall the 'donation' procedure. The cup they had given me looked dreadfully small. I don't mention that as a way to exaggerate the size of my masculinity (just say 'penis'!) but rather because I had never before had to think about the precision of my ejaculation.

NASA is often forced to come up with solutions to assure itself of a shuttle's controlled re-entry. They have experts with doctorates. *I* had no confidence of a controlled entry into this cup, and no scientist on a headset backstage to talk me through it; I had never felt less turned on.

I went to work. I was in a bathroom massaging a flaccid penis, with at least two people in a waiting room on the other side of the door who were aware that I was in a bathroom massaging a flaccid penis. I found one source of inspiration. On the wall behind the toilet hung a seat cover dispenser; on it was the following message:

"To remove seat cover: gently pull up and out."

I read it over and over; up and out, up and out. Five minutes later my donation was complete. I exited the bathroom and made eye contact with my wife who stared with amazement and mouthed 'Already?' across the waiting room, as though she was trying to be clearly understood by a lip reader. At least she wasn't sitting next to my mother. Apparently, she'd only had time to read a couple of pages. For the record: she's a slow reader.

I had placed the receptacle in the *clear* plastic bag provided by the receptionist. When one buys adult magazines at a convenience store, the clerk behind the counter is kind enough to slip it into an opaque bag—they understand customers who purchase such items may want that information kept from the general public. Here, apparently, my cup of sperm was everyone's business. I suppose the clinic is like a pizzeria for sperm donors: There's no point making a pizza box look like anything other than a pizza box since *everyone* here is walking out with a pizza. As for the transparent container, it was now palmed in my hand like a coin in the palm of a magician and pressed against my leg as I smuggled the package back across the waiting room as I would three ounces of heroin. I saw no reason the thirty strangers hanging around the clinic should get even a remote glimpse of a few million of my sperm.

I kept the package well hidden until I made eye contact with the receptionist.

-"All done?" (Already!?)

Screw you, I thought.

I smiled and placed the container on the counter. She tossed it in a plastic basket, slid it through to the lab via a delivery slot in the glass partition and told me I should have the results within 48 hours. I hurried to the door, motioning wide-eyed to my wife that it was time to get the hell out of there and to try to make the best of the day. Maybe go for a beer? Or play in traffic.

§

"Men are such babies."

I hear that a lot. It is often followed by the following justification: If men had to give birth, they couldn't handle the pain and discomfort. The same is said with regard to menstru-ation. It seems that men can never complain about having to shave daily for work without being reminded that that level of inconvenience pales in comparison to the intrusion of a monthly period and the pain of menstrual cramps. Sure, men will wince and exhale in pain if they get jostled in the testes, but it's nothing compared to the pain of childbirth.

How could I tell my wife that being sequestered in a bathroom and masturbating into a cup while strangers waited for my sperm sample made me feel violated in a way I never thought possible? How can a man talk about feelings of violation when globally women are subjected to far worse, far more frequently? Yet, that's how I felt: shamed and embarrassed.

After "the donation," I would look for an outlet through which I could share my experience. Consistently, the mere mention of "sperm test" elicited an identical response: People smiled or giggled or sat gape-mouthed. Everyone assumed that it was something a man would love to do as much as possible because, after all, for men it was all about the orgasm, right? Each time I dared mention the word "embarrassment" or "humiliated" or "violated," the answers would be the same:

-"Yeah? Try getting your period every month."

-"Yeah? Try giving birth."

-"Try living with stretch marks."

Most of all, my wife's story would follow: Try having fluid injected past your cervix and dealing with *that* pain while a large machine takes photographs of your innards.

They were right; all I had done was masturbate.

Then I found out I would have to do the whole thing all over again.

§

The results from the first set of tests revealed "low motility."

-"Mobility?" I asked the urologist.

-"No, *motility*."

Motility is apparently a qualitative measurement of your sperm and refers to what percentage of your sperm are moving as well as the quality of the sperm making up that group.[1]

I was afraid to ask if I had the Flash Gordon of sperm, only too few of them or an army of millions who couldn't find their heads with their tails.

Either way, Dr. Sperm said proper procedure was to perform a second test and compare those results to the first one. The original results from the clinic were not indicative, since the motility level was *borderline acceptable*. I was half-empty or half-full; I wasn't sure which. All I knew is I would be handed another empty plastic container at another clinic (hopefully one with seat covers on the washroom wall).

Since more than a month had elapsed between the first donation and my follow-up doctor's appointment, I would need to provide *two* new samples. The reason being in order to achieve an accurate result, two samples should be taken approximately three days apart; that way they are from the same "batch" of sperm. The easiest way to proceed with the new round of spermograms (doesn't that sound like it describes a sperm showing up at your door with a balloon, singing a show tune?) was to donate once at home into a sealed cup 72 hours prior to our next appointment at the hospital with the fertility specialist; I would then donate again at the hospital itself. Why not? We always had an hour or so to kill in the hospital waiting room; why spend that

---

1   http://www.americanfertility.com/services/male.php

time reading *People*, sipping coffee and watching CNN when I could instead be masturbating? It's not like there was anyone to talk to.

Part of the problem with never discussing masturbation casually around a dinner table is it makes donating sperm at home in your own bathroom more awkward than it needs to be. My wife waited in the bedroom opposite the bathroom, too giggly and curious to be anywhere else. I couldn't handle her being in there with me, maybe even helping out; it felt too awkward. Besides space was scarce; our bathroom also housed our washer and dryer. Again, I wasn't the only one in the room agitating and gyrating. Isn't it romantic?

What was so embarrassing? What was so funny? What was so humiliating? Nothing. When you looked at the whole situation objectively, nothing was transpiring that wasn't natural sexuality. It was only made to feel unnatural because masturbation is never discussed. It is still taboo. It is one of a long list of things—such as flatulence, pimples and dandruff—that everybody knows exists, yet nobody discusses freely. If we can't summon the courage to make a colleague aware of a piece of spinach stuck between their teeth, how will we ever stop hiding our masturbation?

At the hospital, the 'donation room' looked like something out of a detox center. It was about 12 feet long by 5 feet wide, equipped with a vinyl-cushioned bed with an elevated headrest and a television. The T.V. wasn't connected to the internal hospital cable system, but rather to an old VCR. It was sitting on a closed cabinet. I eyed the cabinet suspiciously, wondering what viewing materials I might find inside, given the room was part of the fertility clinic.

It was empty.

I also noticed the absence of a box of tissue paper; only coarse brown disposable paper towel on a roll in a dispenser under the sink. I sat for a moment, contemplating how best to proceed. Then my receptacle, my penis and I, found our way to the sink near the paper towels, and away we went. Minutes later: done. Sample number three of three was successfully delivered.

I handed the sample to the receptionist with the same resignation as a man accustomed to watching his favorite team lose and at this point is just showing up for the beer. Repeated clinical masturbation had given me the strength to accept what I could not change.

My wife and I sat down with the OBGYN who was following our case: a charming English fellow. He said my wife's test had come back "normal." He asked if I had the results of my spermogram. I recounted my tale. He spoke to my wife and me with an incredible amount of sympathy and understanding. He reassured us these tests are merely a preliminary stage, and we were not alone in feeling worried and scared at the prospect of not being able to conceive. It was ironic that something that at one point we weren't sure we would ever want, was now the source of such a sense of failure and sadness. He explained that should my sperm test be normal as well, we would then move on to the next step: artificial insemination.

A.I. involves inserting the sperm directly into the woman's uterus through the use of a catheter and syringe. It also carries with it a price tag of several hundred dollars per attempt. Dr. Baby explained the chances of reproducing with A.I. is about one in three, and three attempts are all they will try before moving on to in vitro fertilization, which carries with it a greater risk and a price tag in the thousands.

He said that, for right now, we should continue trying naturally, and we should visit him again at the beginning of my wife's next menstrual cycle to proceed with the first step of A.I.

But the next time we saw Dr. Baby, it would be for an entirely different reason.

· HONESTY TIP FOR THE iDAD ·

Force yourself to discuss things that make you feel uncomfortable. It's the first step toward healthy communication between yourself, your partner and your children.

BACK FROM THE FUTURE

From Blog to Book

I

Inspired by the MenGetPregnantToo.com Post: Men Are
Allowed to Complain! – Published: July 6, 2011

Prior to becoming a father, I had never really undergone a painful medical procedure (I don't remember my circumcision, nor do I remember the hangover that followed). However, as I age, I seem to be more and more often blessed with the opportunity to lie my body on an examination table for further review. Since this is *What Do I Do While You're Pregnant?* and not *Men Whine About Medical Procedures* I'll focus on only one such occasion—by far the most uncomfortable—the cystoscopy. I feel compelled to briefly explain the procedure in order for the context of my point to be fully appreciated:

A tube is threaded through the urethra into the bladder. The bladder is then filled with liquid until it expands to full capacity. (Have you ever been out for drinks with friends and then stuck in a traffic jam on the way home? Or been on a road trip, polished off a few large coffees and found yourself 45 miles from a rest stop? Remember how painful that was?) The doctor now clamps your urethra shut by squeezing your penis while muttering something about it "not being much longer." Throughout this experience a team of eager students huddle in a corner craning their necks to get a better view of your groin. (The best part was when the medical professor pointed out the following useful information to the students: "See how his toes are clenching? That's a classic sign of severe discomfort." I'll show you severe discomfort, Dr. Know-it-all.)

Once the bladder is fully distended, the tube is withdrawn (back through the urethra) and a scope (with camera!) is inserted in its place—kinda like the one used in the first *Mission Impossible* movie: the one they slip through the grate enabling them to scope the vault.

With this camera, the urologist (I don't know if urologist should be capitalized; all I know is he didn't deserve to be) can examine my bladder interior, as well as the functionality of a couple of sphincters in the region. (Yes, I know! I also thought we had only one, but there are more than fifty sphincters in the human body!) As he looks through the camera he is manipulating with one hand; with the other hand he gradually releases the pressure on my urethra (a euphemism for 'no longer squeezing my penis'), allowing me to slowly evacuate the liquid. During this painfully slow emergency evacuation, he keeps hypnotically repeating "Just relax. Not much longer. Just relax."

I recounted this experience to a few of my male friends in the presence of their female wives. The men unanimously cringed and physically withdrew into their chairs the longer I spoke. But while I did, on one occasion, get a sympathetic reaction from a woman (my wife, exhibiting a "reason-I-married-her" #143 in a series), the other reactions all resembled each other. I wrote about them, along with a similar reaction to a friend's prostate exam, in this post:

"Try getting your period every month."

A family friend recently underwent a prostate exam. He commented how uncomfortable he felt lying on his side while someone's finger snuck in the back door. He didn't complain it was painful, he didn't miss work and he didn't refuse to empty the dishwasher. He said, "I felt uncomfortable."

The response from the woman he was with: "Try having a baby."

On behalf of Men, let me clear the air with some grand concessions: Pregnancy and birth bring with them back pain, swollen feet, nausea, interruptions in sleep patterns, horrible cramping, loss of appetite, muscle strain—both internal and external—resulting from hosting a growing human being for nine months and then expelling it through an opening previously only used for much more meager purposes, wild hormone changes and a host of other symptoms men will never fully appreciate since we will (most likely) never experience childbirth. Granted, acknowledged, agreed and confessed.

Now, can you allow us that it's uncomfortable having a finger up our ass? Especially someone else's.

During my wife's pregnancy, I felt intimidated to not express too strongly feelings of physical or emotional discomfort. I realized that with her undergoing such a massive physical transformation, my expressions might be misconstrued as attempts at competition for attention. Now that the experience is years behind us, I realize pregnancy is the gift that keeps on giving. In many circles, even a nine-month cystoscopy would be met with scepticism by those who have been through childbirth.

To them, I say: "Look, I'm doing my best to keep up, all right? I may never push a watermelon through a pigeon hole, but I've had a doctor scope my urethra. That's *got* to be worth something."

CHAPTER 4

Only 280 Days to Go

Assuming overtime at the Super Bowl is the pinnacle
of a man's capacity for excitement.

The artificial insemination procedure coincides with the woman's ovulation cycle. Our instructions were to report back to the OBGYN's office as soon as my wife begins her next period. In the meantime we continued with our homework. At least she never suggested I get a tutor. Sex on Monday. No sex on Tuesday. Sex on Wednesday. No Sex on Thursday. Day on. Day off. Only a couple of more weeks before we head back to The Fertility Clinic—a sterile place with a sterile name.

We watched days come and go until finally, 28 days later, my wife's period was to begin. It conjured images of a conductor in front of an orchestra, as though we would wake on the twenty-eighth morning and my wife's Ovulation Maestro would tap his baton and…voilà! The Period would begin.

But it didn't.

It's a funny thing, eagerly awaiting the arrival of a period. What would normally be a regular day becomes filled with tension and mystique. There are few things that will send your adrenaline into overdrive more than a phone call received at work saying, "Ummm, so, I didn't get my period yesterday."

My heart started racing; does this mean what I think it means? Don't get too excited, now.

-"Have you been late before?" I asked.

I wasn't sure what answer I was looking for. If she told me yes, she had been late before, my day would suddenly take a very anti-climactic turn. If, however, she were to admit that she is rarely late, it could mean that THIS COULD BE THE DAY!

-"Sometimes, but not often," she answered.

Huh? What do I do with that?

I can remember when I first became sexually active. I was just shy of 19 years old—young enough to be stupid, but old enough to be terrified of a girl who says she is a day late. Eighteen is a very dangerous age for a young man; you're beginning to learn some long-term lessons of life, but your testosterone still has more control over your body than does your conscious mind. And when you're rolling around with a girl who is willing to go all the way, resistance is futile. I would never have imagined that that feeling would be turned on its head in adulthood. Here I was, praying for a late period and having the bottom drop out of my gut every time the period came, knowing it meant at least another month's delay and homework before fatherhood.

We both talked each other down, like coaches on a team: "Don't get excited. Let's wait another day or two. It probably doesn't mean anything." Yadda, yadda, yadda. We knew what we were thinking: WOOHOO!!!! A BABY! But still, we behaved very sensibly for the next thirty-six hours. Once a day-and-a-half had passed and no period came, we knew it was time to consult *the stick*.

§

The day before our wedding, my in-laws gave us a Dr. Spock book and an Early Pregnancy Test Kit. My extend-ed family is about as subtle as the Washington Monument is androgynous. Ironically, the gift, which had raised my ire on my wedding weekend (*can we at least pay the caterer before we supply you with grandchildren!?*), would now serve me quite well during my little crisis. I dug the E.P.T. out of the armoire, and my wife went to the washroom (*NOW* who's in the bathroom alone running tests?).

The instructions specify that once the stick is "moist" (anything can be given a touch of elegance in the hands of the right marketing expert), the observers are to wait two minutes before expecting a result.

Let's take a moment to admit to all those silly games we play with ourselves while assuming no one is aware of them. For example: 'If I get this piece of paper into the trash basket from the other side of the room, I'll ask the boss for the raise' or 'If I flip this coin and get three heads in a row, it means she'll call me for a second date' or 'If I don't peek at the E.P.T. stick during the two-minute wait period, the test result will be positive.'

We huddled like college students in a hallway, with the stick having a moment to itself on top of the bathroom vanity. We could have stood over it, but suddenly we firmly believed the adage: "A watched pot never boils," ergo: An observed E.P.T. stick never changes its hue.

Tick-Tock, Tick-Tock. Two minutes waiting for a pregnancy test is exactly like the feeling you get when you leave on a road trip headed for the beach and run into four hours of traffic. It was enough to make me want to scream. We literally stood there looking at the seconds hand on my watch.

Two minutes was up. Into the bathroom we went.

The Stick lay there like a sentry. I don't know why, but I expected it would have crawled out the window simply to deny us an answer. We looked down to see a little blue +. After quadruple checking the instructions, it was confirmed: We were pregnant. Yes, *We*. At least we were pretty sure we were.

§

I am definitely the more 'particular' person in the relationship. I like to know what's next, what we're doing this weekend, who's coming over, how long the visit is going to last, and then, what we're doing after that. If we aren't doing anything this weekend, I like to know that as well so I can plan for doing nothing at all. I call this trait 'particular;' some may refer to it in a less politically correct (however perhaps more appropriate) fashion as 'anal.' Maybe it is because of this character trait I happened to notice the expiration date on the E.P.T. box. Woops. It was two months expired. I expect my in-laws would be sorely disappointed to find it took us beyond the shelf life of their gift to become pregnant. However, it did not change the fact that, according to the instructions on this box, this device was no longer reliable.

Thanks to having stared at my watch diligently for the last two minutes, we knew it was just shy of 11 p.m., which meant that the local pharmacy was still open. There was a short but intense discussion about whether I was being too 'particular'; but when it comes to confirming a pregnancy, the word 'assume' should not be in the cards. Off I went.

I bought two more. One can never be careful (anal) enough. Second test: Positive. Third test a day later: Positive. We were pregnant…for sure.

Within seconds, I hit an emotional high. I couldn't believe it. The metaphor of a bull in a china shop would have been an accurate description. The difference between me and the bull is that I was a bull who was absolutely terrified of breaking anything. I wanted to pick my wife up off her feet and swing her around like a tetherball—but I didn't want to hurt the baby. I wanted to pop the cork on a battle of champagne—but I didn't want to hurt the baby (and we didn't have any champagne). I wanted to blast the soundtrack from "Rocky III"—but I didn't want to hurt the baby (or lead my wife to believe she had made a horrible mistake vis-à-vis her choice of husband). So we smiled, we hugged, we kissed and then did so again for a good half-hour. And then all we could do was go to bed.

Sure.

Sleep.

Easier said than done.

The machine gun thought process started up all over again: Boy or girl? Healthy or not? To tell people or not? Twins or not? Easy pregnancy ahead or not? Better get to reading those books. Better get to doing those exercises. Better start watching that diet. Better start learning how to keep a secret. Better find a way to kill time until the next morning since all we wanted to do now was call the doctor. All we wanted to do was TELL SOMEBODY!

But we couldn't call anyone…it was late; it was time for bed, again. And so we lay there and analyzed our future—and the child who would share it—over and over again, until the hospital switchboard opened.

I think one of the things I am learning as I grow older is I am not as special and unique as I would like to think I am. I am never the first one to experience something; I can never trump the experts with my life experience; I have never told a story that has made the room go silent. So I don't know why I was surprised when the reaction at the fertility clinic switchboard to the announcement that my wife was pregnant was met with no more enthusiasm than that of someone who had been told the city bus was running on schedule this afternoon (all I did was show up at that stop every second day, after all). I don't know what else I expected. This clinic has been around for fifty years, seeing fifty patients a day. Minus closures for statutory holidays, that works out to more than eight-hundred-thousand patients. Surely we were not the first to conceive naturally. But it was ME, dammit!

Anyway, polite congratulations were given, and we were given an appointment for our first ultrasound three months later. Three months. That famous first trimester when you are keeping the whole thing a secret from everyone, when you have yet to see a picture of your unborn child and you must refer to it as "it" since you still do not know the sex. For the guy, all there is to do is keep your mouth shut and watch your wife experience stress and morning sickness and colds and headaches for which she is not permitted to take any medication; hardly a great first ten steps out of the starting blocks.

So there we sat: reading the books, examining the charts, holding hands and talking about parenthood amongst ourselves for a month. Of course, after promising we would tell no one, we each admitted to the other that we had each secretly snuck off and shared the news with our closest friends, each of us believing the other would be upset at the betrayal. But the other wasn't. The other understood that it is unnatural to keep information of this scale to yourself for longer than a minute or two. Still, the secret went no further than us and those two friends.

The *idea* of telling no one else is interesting. Our reason was, by-and-large, due to our not wanting to have to give family members grim updates should something go medically awry. However, I think we both knew that if we ended up losing the baby—or my wife was hospitalized due to an emergency situation—we would both inform our families, anyway. But the benefit for me of keeping the news within the household was it allowed us to digest the news on our own terms. It delayed the suggestions about how to handle the early stages of pregnancy, as well as the questions about what we are or are not experiencing emotionally and physically. It put off people requesting an inventory of what we do or do not already have at home for the baby. It kept at bay inquiries about our hopes for the child's sex, and after whom we are or are not naming the baby, and so on. It allows you keep people in the dark without fear of being blindsided by questions you are not prepared—or willing—to answer. So as much as I was bursting with excitement while listening to the hamster in my head running its wheel into the ground, I was equally happy being Superman in our little fortress of solitude.

Superman, who freaked out when his wife started spot-bleeding.

§

The first day we were pretty sure it was nothing; a little blood. The Good (self-help) Books said not to worry about a little blood. The Good Books also throw in that famous caveat that we would come to know so well:

"While 'X' is perfectly normal—and seen in 'X' percentage of cases—persistent or unusually painful 'X' is reason enough to see a physician."

This 'X' represents any sign or symptom you've never seen before. During your first pregnancy, that's all of them. How long before a symptom is 'persistent'? What threshold of pain is 'unusual'? They don't say. Thanks for nothing. I need a chart!

A few days went by, and the bleeding did not stop. Finally, a merciful nurse told us to come in for a checkup, preceded by the reassuring statement, which is more the cornerstone of the medical profession than is the Hippocratic oath: "I'm sure it's nothing".

After an examination, our mild-mannered—wonderful-ly British—Dr. Baby explained that spot bleeding was often caused by the fertilized egg implanting itself into the soft wall of the uterus. When you think about the science of this stuff, it really is absolutely mind-blowing. Not only the transforma-tion of this sperm and egg into a human, but a human being's capacity—through study and technology—to be able to un-derstand and identify so specific a problem. To be sure it was

nothing more serious, he would send us for an immediate ultrasound. It took everything I had not to scream like a
teenager: "AWESOME!" we were going to get a look at our
kid…'It.'

My wife lay down on the table, the monitor was rolled over
and I took my dutiful position as Husband-Hand-Holder by the
side of the gurney. It was just like on TV:

Firstly: "This will feel a little cold."

Then: "Just relax."

Followed by: "You'll feel a little pressure."

Husband-Hand-Holders must sit quietly and nod and listen
and hand-hold and stroke hair while every fiber of their being
wants to yell: "SHOW US THE DAMN PICTURE!"

While this may sound insensitive, remember I have been
given the biggest news of my life. It will shape the course of
my future and yet I physically feel no change. To compensate
for this numbness, I have supportively asked of my wife "How
are you feeling?" three times a day since conception. This is my
first brush with the reality of the situation. The first time I will
see physical proof of my impending fatherhood (E.P.T. dipstick
aside). 'Excited' is this moment's great understatement.

When we were kids, my father ran a business dealing in
the first generation of home computers. He brought home a
Texas Instruments PC, complete with an audio cassette onto
which you saved your work. We also owned a newly minted
version of "Pong"—a black and white game with the two
rectangular paddles that deflected a square ball around the screen
accompanied by a soundtrack of various beeps and bops. The

resolution of this ultrasound was nearly half as good as that 1976 Texas Instruments video game.

-"There's your cervix," the technician explained. I leaned in to get a better look.

-"The dark area is your uterus," she continued. I physically moved my chair even closer to the screen, worried I was the only one in the room not understanding what I was seeing.

-"And in the center, you will notice a flashing light." She gestured. Let me guess, that's the opponent's ball trying to score on my net.

-"That's the heartbeat," she clarified.

I froze.

Clearly we could all see what looked like a pin-sized signal beacon from a miniscule one-hundred-watt light bulb flashing twice per second at the center of a dark area.

The heartbeat.

My body became covered with gooseflesh. The skin on my arms and around my head began constricting as though it was too small for my body. I leaned towards the monitor...closer... closer. Nothing was said for what seemed like hours, as everything in that room was happening in slow motion for me. I was unconsciously squeezing my wife's hand so tightly it had gone white and numb. I am trying not to hyperbolize the memory, but it is difficult to express it in any other way than this: I was witnessing a miracle. One single sperm measuring one-six-hundredth of a millimeter had found its way into one single egg and had in less than two months produced a heartbeat. There was the beginning of whoever would be borrowing my car sixteen years from now.

I cried.

I need to briefly digress.

One of the obstacles the human race should make a point of overcoming—other than the shame of masturbation—is men feeling the need to avoid crying in public. Even worse is the need to LIE about crying. The whole thing is just plain weird.

Now, back to our story: I cried.

I cried for joy. I cried as a release of nervous tension I didn't even know was there. I cried because our baby was alive. I cried because my wife was crying, and I cried because everything going on in that room, at that moment, made cosmic sense.

I am glad that I took those few moments, and the couple of weeks after that first examination, to really *feel* what was happening. I rolled around in my excitement like a puppy on a new rug. I was glad I did not rush past the experience of finding out that, after all that time and effort and research and hope, things had turned out exactly as they should. All was normal and everyone was healthy. I was glad because it prepared me for the terrifying news to come.

· EMOTIONAL TIP FOR THE iDAD ·

Allow yourself to experience The Moment. Stop worrying about what you *should* feel and instead, embrace what you *are* feeling.

CHAPTER 5

What if Our Perfect Baby is Not So Perfect?

As a part of his role as father-to-be, as life partner to a pregnant woman and as a generally decent human being, a husband's job is to make sure his wife is as comfortable as possible during her pregnancy. This is done with whatever creature comforts are available to a layman: kindness, favorite foods and massages are but a few. As far as monitoring her physical health and ensuring all is well with the fetus, that must be entrusted to the medical profession. In addition to a second ultrasound three months into the pregnancy, there was a battery of blood tests and urine tests and scales to step on and forms to fill in. Then there were the 'hands-on' exams: feeling, looking, measuring, squeezing and poking. The results always came back normal. Normal, normal, normal. So, why should we choose to examine this pregnancy any further? For much the same reason mountain climbers risk their lives: because it's there; because we can. Much like the group who rebuilt the Six-Million-Dollar Man 30 years ago, we have the technology.

Pregnancies become games of chance and statistics. What are the risks versus benefits of undertaking—or choosing not to participate in—any given course of treatment? There are so many evaluations to make, it becomes a game of fill-in-the-blank: Don't smoke because it increases the chance of ____; don't drink because it increases the chance of___; eat well because the baby will have a better chance of___; etc. And there is the constant warning of the dark truth: "One in three women loses a baby. But, don't worry; you seem to be doing fine."

Most babies who are miscarried are lost during the first trimester, although there are exceptions. After every round of tests, there is encouragement from the medical community that always comes with an asterisk. "Chances are that—with the results we've seen on the standard tests—your baby will be perfectly healthy, although there is no way to know for sure until you're further along."

You really can make yourself crazy. And if you talk to enough pregnant people (and their husbands), you'll notice that some of them *are* crazy. They become crazy with worry and crazy with analysis. People can become obsessed with research and numbers and percentages and statistics. My wife and I always believed that, at some point, the stress you put yourself through by worrying and researching negates any minor positive changes you might make during the pregnancy as a result of your Google searches. If you believe—as we did—that your baby has the capacity to feel your stress, you'll convince yourself to relax and save yourself a world of trouble.

So why then did we, after being told all of the exams indicated a perfectly healthy pregnancy, decide to go to a private clinic for *one more test*? Because of two words. The two words that will drive every parent, and parent-to-be, up a wall:

What if?

What if we are the 'one' in the 'one out of every million'? *What if* what happened to that woman in Iceland we read about online a couple of months ago happens to me? *What if* I could have prevented it and didn't? *What if* something turns out to be my fault?

What if? What if? What if?

So when the hospital told us we could be further reassured

of a healthy pregnancy by paying for a triple screen at a private clinic, the question really became, What if we don't and something happens?

What if?

So we took the test.

§

The triple screen is also called the AFP test. This test gives the lab the ability to look at a sample of AFP—Alpha-Fetoprotein: a protein passed from the fetus's liver into the mother's bloodstream. This can flag all sorts of potential trouble: from physical defects in the growth of the baby, to Down Syndrome. The test claims to catch most things that can possibly go wrong and yet would normally remain undetected during a pregnancy. For a couple of hundred dollars, we went ahead with the test. We knew we would either have our minds put further at ease or be driven to despair.

When they phoned us with the results, we realized we were in the latter group.

The analogy of being punched in the stomach is used frequently to describe how one feels after receiving bad news. Upon receiving the results of the triple screen, I knew why. My wife got off the phone pale and shaking, barely able to speak. She was not hysterical, but there was sadness in her face that I had never seen before. And then she told me:

-"The lab called to say that the test has shown a higher than normal risk for Down Syndrome."

I was sitting on the bed and had no idea what to do with

myself.

-"Oh." Was all I could manage.

I crawled over, took her hands and we sat together crying quietly for a while. I think I managed a few stock lines: "It'll be okay." "The test could still be wrong." "Even with these results, the odds are all in our favor." All the standards. I was the Frank Sinatra of husbandly support. The only person in the room who believed in me less than my wife was me. How could we have come this far only to have this happen?

I know many people have children with Down Syndrome. Parents have all kinds of children. Children of all kinds are loved by many, and rightfully so. That being said, I believe no one on the planet would respond to this news differently from the way we did. It is not a moment which lends itself to rational judgment and detached evaluation; it is a time taken over by hearts and feelings and instinct. It is visceral, not intellectual, and it is out of our control.

Eventually the immediate grieving passed. Not the grieving for a physical loss but the grieving for an idea. It was grieving for a belief that was stronger for us than anything else thus far in our lifetime: the belief that, despite what all the literature warned us about, nothing was going to go wrong with this pregnancy.

Soon we realized there was a conversation to be had.

The conversation was filled with euphemism for life's ugly side: "We should find out what our options are." "What if the baby has special needs?" and "What kind of life will this child have?"

It was all smoke and mirrors for what was not being said: Do we or don't we want to have an abortion?

§

Our first job was to find out what we could about Down Syndrome. The two of us looked across the table at each other and, with our laymen backgrounds, carefully expressed our feelings about having a child with special needs.

Neither of us had any firsthand experience with Down's or any other form of genetic disorder. I was embarrassed to realize that my only experience with anything other than a 'normal' life was through the news media and various forms of fiction. My only frame of reference for Down Syndrome was TV sitcoms and after school specials. In each case, the Down Syndrome child was portrayed as happy, playful, eager, polite and respectful of everyone.

I have been around enough children, and was one myself once, to know that no child is perfect, and all parents at one time or another (sometimes suddenly, from one minute to the next) want to bury their heads in their pillows, pull their hair out and scream at the wall. I was not naïve—I realized that raising a special neeeds child would come with the same challenges as raising any baby plus other complications I was not yet aware of. But, at that moment, in the first hours after receiving the news that our baby may have a genetic defect, I was prepared to deal with the challenge of the unknown. I was telling myself that after all the excitement I had at the prospect of becoming a father, I could not imagine opting for terminating the pregnancy.

My wife was more skeptical. Her thought process was less foolhardy. She was lending more weight to the emotional and physical demands a Down Syndrome child could represent. She was brave enough to ask: Do I have enough strength, stamina, conviction and patience to undertake the responsibility of raising a child with Down Syndrome? What if the personal demands are far more than we are prepared for? She was not sure she had it in her to give. At that moment, while I was disappointed, I also asked myself if there was a chance I saw raising a child with a genetic defect as a test, a personal badge of honor. Was it something I was pushing myself to do just to say that I could? I was in my early thirties; she was nearly forty. What would become of our baby twenty years from now? Our family trees were not Redwoods; we had few relatives who were viable options to takeover caring for our baby when we no longer could.

I began to see the situation as lose/lose: If we went ahead with the abortion, and were not able to conceive again, I would be forever regretful. If we conceived again, and the same tests produced the same results, would we abort again? And again? When do we give up? And, if we kept the baby and found years down the road that our relationship, and lives, were suffering because the situation was more difficult than we imagined, would my wife be resentful for having capitulated?

I wondered how long I could stare blankly at the wall until I was forced to make a decision. We were in the dining room, sitting in silence, each waiting for the other to make the first move.

Our first move was to slide over to the computer and log onto the web.

§

The internet's great blessing is that it's a great tool for an individual not yet ready to share information with flesh-and-blood human beings. It is anonymity exemplified. While it unfortunately will teach you how to build bombs and poison cats, it will also give you access to topical information without having to let another human being in on your secret. It is a great cave in which to crawl around and gather information on topics perceived largely as taboo.

One of the challenges of taboo topics is: Open internet conversations and forum discussions on those topics can be monopolized by fringe groups. Regular folks are sometimes so busy denying that unfortunate things happen to them that when those things do occur, there are no other regular folks to talk about it with. Also, community forums are the road rage of online conversation. Since everyone can present themselves through an alias and an avatar, there are no real consequences to being rude and hurtful. Often these trolls scare off users who are just looking to participate in intelligent, helpful conversation.

Despite that, I went online hoping to gather firsthand information about what life was like with a Down Syndrome child. The websites seemed divided into two categories: medical information—lists of the causes, symptoms and complications of the genetic defect; and religious—church-going parents extolling the virtues of their Down's child, regardless of medical difficulties. This latter group professed how precious their families were to them and how they could not imagine life without their son or daughter.

What I found troublesome about the latter group is they

had no examples of what day-to-day life was like with a Down Syndrome child. There was no mention of what work would be involved in managing the medical care of someone who, by all accounts, is experiencing some range of complications included on the lists within the *first* group of sites: mild to moderate mental retardation, congenital heart defect, pulmonary hypertension, poor hearing and vision that require constant monitoring during a child's development, thyroid problems, intestinal abnormalities, seizure disorders, respiratory problems, obesity, an increased susceptibility to infection and a higher risk of childhood leukemia.[2]

I was not looking for any specific case study; any real-life essay would do. Other than a choir echoing the general joys of parenting—regardless of the health of the child—no parents I could find were writing openly of their experiences with a Down Syndrome child. Predominantly, the information available told me—very non-specifically—that everything would be fine. Then my eye would wander back to that infamous list; that list of potential problems, each representing potential stress, anguish and possible regret. But to what degree? There was no way to know. Understandably, parents with special-needs children are not going to easily admit—especially not to an online forum—that they have second thoughts. It must be a hard enough job parenting a difficult child without also allowing yourself to entertain the thought that life would be easier without that child. That admission must be torture. But is it occasionally the truth?

We called the doctor's office, informed them of the results of the triple screen and asked for an appointment to discuss op-

---

2   http://www.kidshealth.org/parent/medical/genetic/down_syndrome.html

tions.

§

Question: Doctor, what conclusions should we draw from these test results?

Answer: One option is undergoing another test, which will be conclusive: an amniocentesis.

Of course, another test.

The ambiguity about the health of our unborn child can be all but erased with the help of a long needle inserted through the woman's abdomen and into the amniotic sac—hopefully avoiding the fetus—to remove a sample of amniotic fluid. The fluid, once sent to the lab, will reveal with much more accuracy the health of the baby.

Okay, we thought, let's do it. We told the doctor we would like to have the test done, and upon receiving the test results, decide whether we would keep the baby.

Statistics reared their ugly head again. Dr. Baby explained the test itself carries a one in two-hundred chance of miscarriage. This means that the amnio should only be done if we are considering an abortion. If we think we will end up wanting to keep the child regardless, it is not recommended we put the fetus through the stress of the procedure.

We recounted to him our dilemma; we told him of the dead ends we ran into when we tried to investigate what life would be like with a Down Syndrome child.

At first, he performed his medical duty and remained frustratingly neutral. He explained that it is not a doctor's right to project onto parents whether they should keep a child. It is a very personal decision and one that will affect our life as a couple, forever, not to mention the dynamic of a family for generations to come.

We pressed. And pressed. Our point was this: We felt too uninformed and too inexperienced with Down's to be able to make an educated decision, especially one that carries with it such weight and consequences. Eventually, he admitted what the websites would not: Life with a Down's child *can*—although not necessarily *will*—be very difficult. Medical problems can send you to the hospital frequently, even several times a week. The child's development can often include several operations, as well as the varying degrees of the complications we found in our research. Finally, there was a reluctant, soft-spoken admission that he did have patients with Down's children who revealed to him that, given the opportunity a decade ago, would have chosen to avail themselves of the modern tests that are now available in order to have made a more informed decision. One can only imagine the pain they must have felt saying those words out loud to another human being.

After moments of silence, we said we would like to go ahead with the amnio as soon as possible.

§

The amniocentesis introduced us to a medical Catch-22: The further along the fetus is in its development, the more accurate the test results. This meant, after receiving the results of the triple screen three months into the pregnancy, we would have to wait another month before subjecting the baby to a procedure that may prove fatal.

This also meant keeping the pregnancy quiet from our families even longer. We agreed we did not want to tell our parents of the growing grandchild only to have to immediately put a hold on their elation to tell them that the baby may have Down Syndrome. And we certainly did not want to subject them to the emotional trauma of knowing that if the condition exists, we do not intend to keep the baby. Our choice would be a source of devastation for them for the rest of their lives. Dealing with their heavyheartedness, while trying to manage our own regret, would prove to be insufferable.

One of the most difficult realizations for us was that by the time we received the test results from the amnio, the pregnancy would be far enough along that—should we decide not to keep the baby—my wife would actually have to go through labor. I am not a religious person, but I knew the only thought I would have while watching my wife go through labor to give birth to a still-born child we were making a conscious decision not to keep would be *forgive me.*

We each shared the latest development with our respective close friends, who had by now become our unofficial family therapists and then sat for a month and waited for another test, which would again determine the course of the rest of our lives.

Observing the attitude of the staff at the hospital's test center, I felt like I was a client at a hotel. They were friendly, warm, courteous and very aware that the people in front of them were bracing themselves for a day that could possibly include some very bad news.

We were brought into an exam room, my wife on a gurney

and me, once again, in my chair, dutifully holding a hand. The ultrasound machine stood like a robot, which, for the moment, had been switched off. Unlike the last ultrasound, the tone of the room was decidedly more somber and quiet. The doctor came in; she was in her early thirties. When you are a teenager and visit a doctor who is in her 30s, she is clearly a person of authority; she might as well be 65. When you are in your early 30s, visiting a doctor who is in *her* early 30s and is armed with an 8-inch syringe, you are tempted to ask her to produce some form of accreditation. She smiled, introduced herself and confidently stated: "I will be performing your amnio today."

Would I like fries with that?

I don't like needles. I have attempted to donate blood on four separate occasions and passed out during each of them. I also fainted once while visiting my mother at work in a neonatal unit and twice during a class at college where the topic was "psychic surgery." The college video showed a "surgeon" in some remote country appearing to remove spoiled body parts from someone's abdomen with his bare hands while leaving no scar. I didn't for a second believe the surgery was real, but there was enough fake blood on the screen to make me drop to the classroom floor. In a poor attempt at saving face in front of my teenage classmates, I promised the teacher I could make my own way to the school nurse. I passed out again in the hallway. So the prospect of watching a doctor slowly push a needle into my wife while carefully trying her best to avoid our unborn baby made me feel anxious, to say the least. My wife thought I was holding her hand, but little did she know that she was actually holding mine.

The doctor began to palpate the area while looking at the ultrasound monitor (the cyborg had come to life). I asked her what she was looking for. She replied that she was looking for a pocket of empty space where the amniotic fluid was and the fetus was not. That sounded very logical to me. I said no more. She looked and felt and prodded and poked and finally said:

-"There we go, that will do. Now I'm going to ask you not to move."

More needless words were never spoken. I wasn't sure if she was talking to me or to my wife, but it didn't matter— I was frozen. On the monitor, I saw the tip of the needle, represented by a fine white line against the black background of the computer monitor, sliding down into the uterus. I suddenly told myself this was a moment in my life for which I needed to be fully present. I was not going to look away, or hold my breath and wait for it to pass. Nor was I going to pass out in the middle of a high-risk medical procedure. I forced myself to look at the needle itself, and to see firsthand what my wife was being subjected to. When she asked me what it looked like, I was NOT going to answer, "I don't know; I wasn't watching."

The doctor's hand, holding the needle, seemed to have a slight tremor, which made me nervous, though this was no time to express concern. The image was almost surreal. The needle entering the abdomen seemed as though it was not actually puncturing the skin, but collapsing against it. The image on the monitor of the white line getting longer and longer seemed like some sort of optical illusion. Yet a moment later, the plunger was drawn back and the needle slid neatly out of my wife's body. The procedure was done.

I was relieved that, at that moment, everything seemed to be normal: There was no blood; the doctor said the procedure had gone normally; my wife seemed fine; the ceiling was still up and the floor was still down. All was well for a minute or two, and then we both remembered the laboratory test was only a doorway to the real personal test: What would be the result and how would we cope?

§

The following is a list of suggestions from a pregnancy website which may help while waiting for the results of an amniocentesis:

> "Although it will be difficult, try to keep your mind on other things while you await the results of your testing. Keeping busy at work or with hobbies can help pass the time. You may want to visit with friends, or make a trip to a local salon for a day of pampering."[3]

Right. If you ever want to play an interesting game with yourself while awaiting potentially disastrous test results, do the following: Count how many times you lie to people by answering "Nothing" or "Not Much" when they ask you "What's new?" You'll be amazed at your capacity for deflection.

So we watched TV, walked around the house, rented movies we couldn't focus on, snacked, went to the bathroom more often than we needed to, and went to the office while making concealed fists and chewing on our tongues whenever someone

3   http://www.amazingpregnancy.com/pregnancy-articles/103.html

asked us: "What's new?"

Every time the phone rang, we jumped. Every time it wasn't the hospital, our disappointment came across a little too clearly; people were always telling us we sounded like we weren't happy to hear from them. We lied and told them we were thrilled, just tired; then we quickly found a reason to hang up and leave the line free for someone more important.

Finally, two days later, someone more important called.

-"Hello. This is the hospital test center calling."

-"Yes?"

They thankfully confirmed my wife's identity before divulging our test results.

-"I'm calling to let you know that everything is fine. The test results are negative and the baby is healthy."

-"Um, OK. Thank you."

-"Have a nice day and congratulations."

I must have cried at the news since I'm crying at the memory.

· SUPPORTIVE TIP FOR THE iDAD ·

When saying "Everything will be okay" doesn't seem to work, a hug or just being there may be all that is required.

CHAPTER 6

Open the Floodgates: We're Having a Baby

There is a need in all of us to be *part* of something—to be included, often to the point of seeking a position of privilege over the people around us. For instance: announcing one's knowledge of an upcoming event before others are aware of it, or offering 'helpful advice' to others as a clandestine method of proving you know more about the topic than they do. When someone is pregnant, everyone wants to be the first to know; people have their reasons for believing they are in a position of privilege. Parents believe being such a close relative is reason enough; close friends believe since you often confide things to them you would never tell a parent, they should be the first to know if a child is on the way. Sometimes, even mere acquaintances or colleagues will behave in a manner normally reserved for those who share a much richer personal history with you. Few situations bring out this type of behavior as much as being married and of child-bearing (or in my case child-fathering) age or expecting a child.

As soon as we were married—both of us were already in our thirties—no one hesitated to ask the question; it was thrown at us from all directions like bullets from a machine gun: "When? When are you going to have kids? WhenWhenWhen-WhenWhenWhenWhenWhen?" Sometimes the question comes to you straight-on, as in a job interview; other times it is surreptitiously hidden: "So, what are your plans now that you've tied the knot?" From the point of view of both the person asking the question, as well as the person expected to provide the answer, it's a no-win situation because of the following pitfalls:

Answer #1: "We're trying right away."

Reactions:

-Both men and women will keep after you, now that they know you're trying. Every time they see you—even if it's only been a few days—they will ask: "So?" Nudge, nudge. Wink, wink.

-Men will inevitably look at the hopeful father-to-be with that 'sly-old-dog, look-who's-having-sex-everyday' sneer. You know what? Even if I *am* having sex every day—and it has *yet* to become homework—that sneer is pretty creepy. It suddenly makes me feels like some form of molester; as though I've succeeded in creeping up on my wife and having sex with her without her knowledge.

-There are also those who believe that, despite your age, you shouldn't rush into anything. These are inevitably people for whom parenting (or being married) isn't an entirely pleasant experience. The advice then becomes not to "rush into anything" and to "be sure to take time for yourselves."

Answer #2: We've decided to wait awhile.

Reactions:

-Most people see this as a cue to ask "Wait for what?" Especially when you are already over thirty, you can actually watch them search their own mental thesaurus for a proper manner with which to tell you you're no spring chicken.

-Men, again, will often react like men; something that can be paraphrased as, "Yeah, a little more freedom before you get too tied down. Smart!" As though I've been desperately avoiding marriage and fatherhood, but despite that, the former has caught up with me.

-Almost all people will, as with an admission you're already trying, keep asking every time you see them: "So? Still putting fatherhood on hold?"

Answer #3: We're not sure we want kids.

Reactions:

-This is a beauty. For potential grandparents, the expression is pure shock and awe. They have just been hit in the gut with a demolition ball: they will have no more progeny; the line stops here. Not only that, but they feel they have failed as parents because their children don't want to have children. Death by can opener would be less painful. That's why in this situation, you always lie to parents.

-Other couples who are childless by choice will visibly deflate with relief. It is a rare breed who will admit in public they may not want to be parents, since society as a whole—including your parents, closest friends, movies, TV commercials and magazines—in some way reminds you the world is built around the assumption that people marry and have children. This wish to remain childless suddenly becomes a wonderfully shared secret between you and the other couple. Until of course, one of you changes your mind.

-Guys who already have children often have the funniest reaction. Some look at you as though they never knew *not* having a child was an option, especially if they are dealing with a newborn or toddler. "Waddaya mean, you're not sure you want kids? Does *she* know? What does she think? How'd you talk her out of it? Can I come over on Sunday?"

Whatever the answer, people keep pushing. It is ironic that once a couple becomes pregnant, the standard is to keep the pregnancy quiet for the first three months, the logic being the first trimester is a very fragile time and anything can happen. Especially with developments in technology, parents often want to run a gamut of tests to ensure the health of the baby and to allow time to possibly make what is the most personal decision of their lives. Everyone agrees that allowing the news to be released too soon is a mistake, but everyone keeps hounding you at the press conference looking to make your business their business.

§

But your mind is made up; you are going to try for a baby. The sex works; a baby is on the way. Three months go by; you're ready to share your news with the world, and the world is ready…with its own feedback. Everyone is lined up with versions of how your life is going to change:

-"Say goodbye to sleep."

-"Enjoy your alone time while you have it."

-"Enjoy your couple time while you have it."

-"Nothing will bring you closer than a baby."

-"Nothing tests a marriage more than a child."

-"There goes your freedom, Big Boy."

-"I hope you have a history of great sex. It will make it easier to get used to *no* sex."

George Bernard Shaw was bang-on when he said, "Youth is wasted on the young." When I was five years old, I had my freedom. I went to kindergarten five half-days a week, which included a 30 minute snack-break while watching "The Flintstones", and then I would go home to my ready-made lunch and playtime. I had not yet heard the words 'homework' or 'responsibility.' Since then, life for a middle-class child, adolescent, young adult and eventually adult, is all about choice; we just may not realize it until it's too late. Despite this, people don't treat you as though getting married and having a baby are choices. For some reason, everyone behaves as though these things are unavoidable steps in your life. Maybe it is true that we've figured these things out but aren't willing to admit it yet. Half of marriages end in divorce, and many children have troubled relationships with their parents. Still, we keep hammering away at marriage and parenthood because it is within our human fiber to do so. One of the things that makes it so difficult is that every step of the way people are standing by, waiting to tell you how crazy you are, regardless of the path you choose. It is when you stand up and say you are ready, that you feel ready and committed, when you've read the books and done your research, when you've checked your gut and are prepared to take on 50 percent of the parenting duties because it is what you *want* to do—*that's* when men hint to you that you are stepping into a trap, and women say, "Sure *you're* ready. You're not the one who has to squeeze something the size of a watermelon out of a hole the size of a ping pong ball."

So what is the politically correct procedure for telling individual family member that you are expecting a baby?

There are 'must-do's' that, if not respected, can result in potential disaster. Grandparents-to-be *must* be told face-to-face. This presents a difficult dilemma in our families, which are replete with divorcés. Organizing a get-together with a room full of divorced grandparents is hardly the 'good time' one would associate with announcing such wonderful news. So you must choose who gets invited over first. How do you make sure you can make the rounds of the appropriate relatives before the first one told gets on the phone and starts playing 'operator,' beating you to the punch? What could be worse than calling a grandmother-to-be and having the response be, "Yeah. I know. The other grandmother-to-be told me." Uh-oh.

Generally, among divorced parents, one of the two always remains dominant, either due to proximity, feeling like a kindred spirit, or sheer willpower. In my family that person is my mother. Since on my wife's side, my father-in-law lives 450 miles away with my stepmother-in-law (I know, a lot of hyphens), the fathers unknowingly drew the short straw; the biological grandmoms-to-be would be the first to hear the news.

The stars were aligned; our readiness to announce the pregnancy coincided with Mother's Day. In the Mother's Day cards we included the most recent ultrasound photos. The mothers opened them. There was less excitement in Sydney at the turn of the millennium than there was during the opening of those Mother's Day cards: jumping, screaming, kissing, hugging, all sorts of superlatives—if one can be superlative where a grandchild in concerned.

As much as this book is about illustrating the hidden emotional similarities men and women share during a pregnancy, there is no escaping that sometimes men are uniquely men. My father was thrilled—a huge smile, a big hug and a couple of awkward moments of quiet elation, not quite knowing what to say, other than: "Congratulations." My father-in-law was given the news over the phone, and he had the long distance equivalent of a couple of awkward moments of quiet elation, not quite knowing what to say, other than, "Congratulations." He then passed the phone over to his wife, my stepmother-in-law, who had much more to say. Women: 3; men: 0.

Nature or nurture? What drives the different responses? The men's reaction would drive a woman crazy—how can you be so passive with the discovery of information which carries such weight? It is because of reactions like these that men can be labeled as 'party poopers' and 'sticks in the mud.' Whereas, in men's eyes, the women's reaction is seen as typically... 'womany'—the hysteria, the jumping and the yelling all seem to the man on the other side of the room as over-the-top. Nature or nurture? Have men spent too many generations in a workplace—punching clocks, coming home just in time for supper and avoiding dirty diapers—to let themselves be *really* affected by new life? Or have they just spent too much time watching football and trying to impress each other?

There is not a man on the planet who has not at some point tried desperately to suppress a good cry, be it at a screening of *Schindler's List* or *Brokeback Mountain* or at a wedding or at a funeral or during *Four Weddings and a Funeral.* It is very restrictive to feel so strongly at a certain moment in time only to force yourself to not let the emotion work its way through you because of your need to keep up personal appearances.

Be that as it may, in addition to occasionally stumbling foolishly over a lame explanation when asked by a woman, "How can you not cry at this?" ("...I dunno..."), this guarded, Arnold Schwarzenegger attitude creates an avalanche of awkward moments down life's road as word begins to spread about your little bundle of joy.

As the extended family members begin to learn they are becoming aunts, uncles and cousins-once-removed and as friends learn, they will either be sharing you with your offspring or trying not to admit they may lose touch with you altogether, a man's apparent lack of enthusiasm becomes exponentially more noticeable. All of these people is hearing the news for the first time and, much like watching a rock band on tour, they are elated, exuberant, jumping around the room and, yes, occasionally shrieking. The iDAD, however, is in some respects the aging rock star; we've played the same number-one hit to thousands of people in thousands of towns and must each time remember to muster a proper level of delirium when we raise our fists and shout: "We love you, Chicago!" Or is it Dallas, or New York? I don't remember; I've been on tour for a full month.

Eventually, you get called on it: "You don't seem excited."

Of course I'm excited. I spend nights awake imagining my offspring going to school, getting married, borrowing the car, getting caught making out on my couch and most of all peeing off the changing table and onto the floor. I'm so excited I've already compiled a bible of names: girls' names, boys' names, ethnic names, traditional names, grandparents' names, great-grandparents' names. But, when I am at my 36th stop on my 'We're Pregnant' tour, occasionally I get lazy and tired. Women are much better at keeping up appearances and also better at calling you on appearing nonplussed.

§

Sex, Preferred Sex, Date of Birth and Name. Sex, Preferred Sex, Date of Birth and Name. Sex, Preferred Sex, Date of Birth and Name.

It is the law firm of questions asked of a pregnant couple. It is such a well-polished line of questioning it eventually develops its own ironic frustration. After being asked The Questions for the dozenth time or so, answering them can become tedious. However, The Questions also become so expected that if they are not asked of you, you and your wife are apt to be insulted the person did not care enough about the pregnancy. This is the first crack in the watershed that will eventually end friendships with contemporaries who have no children: Can you manage to at least feign interest in each others' lifestyles?

In order to answer all these questions, you must have researched the answers. The baby's date of birth is usually an easy one, since it is one of the first pieces of information obtained from the doctor's office once the pregnancy is confirmed. As for names, that depends a lot more on the couples' proactivity. We were not very proactive this early into the pregnancy. As far as the sex of the baby, this is a classic clash of ideas that must be worked out between the two parents-to-be. Whether to ask the doctor to reveal the baby's sex during the pregnancy is one of the great divides between the mother and the father and often the first clear capitulation on the part of one of the two parents. In my experience, especially in the case of the first child, the father will concede to the mother's wishes. Most women I know, including my wife, choose to keep the sex a secret until birth. The reason I hear most often is "It is life's only real surprise." I decided if ever there was a time I felt strongly about something, this was it; I owed it to myself to be heard. I wanted the sex of the baby revealed, and here's why:

First of all, unless you live in a subterranean dome alone with a plant, life is full of surprises. Anyone who has gone to school, had a job, had a death in the family, traveled, broken a limb, stubbed a toe, tried to buy groceries on a Sunday or lost a sock in the laundry can tell you all about surprises—never mind the surprises that come with being in a relationship. I have enough surprises in my life. I'd like to know what color to paint the room and to know whether to ask people to buy dresses and to be able to make only one list of names. As I said: I can be a little 'particular.' I like to know what's coming.

Secondly, a woman feels a constant ebb and flow of emotional and physical changes throughout her pregnancy: the fetus grows; her body grows; she experiences sickness, cramps, migraines, fatigue, sleeplessness and mood swings—just to name a few. Within each passing moment, for forty weeks, a woman is flooded with reminders of the baby within her; they are connected all day, every day, everywhere, all the time. And that will be followed by breast feeding. Fathers? We're over here. Hi. How are ya? What can I get ya? The only tool we have to understand the process that is consuming our pregnant wives is to ask: "How are you feeling?" And, if you ask this question too often, even the most well-intentioned wife will occasion- ally have had enough: "Sweetie, I just want to lie quietly for a while." Oh. Okay. I'll be here, wondering how *it* is doing, wondering if *it* is kicking, imagining what life is like for *it* inside the womb.

I did not want five more months of wondering about *it*.

Of course, as long as it is being referred to as *it*, a man will always, by default, refer to *it* as *He*. And since about the time Cyndi Lauper released "Girls Just Wanna Have Fun" (sorry Gloria Steinem, a number one hit on Billboard carries a lot of weight), the man is admonished for assuming *it* is a *He*; so we end up sitting there, rather stupidly, not knowing what to do with ourselves.

I wanted to be able to wonder aloud about my son or my daughter. Knowing the baby's sex would immediately create a connection for me, and my imaginings of my future family would suddenly become more vivid. I offered my wife a compromise: We would ask the doctor to reveal the sex to me alone, and I would then stick the answer in a sealed envelope in my sock drawer. Whenever she felt she couldn't wait any longer, she could feel free to check the findings for herself. She was worried I would slip and, through casual conversation, reveal to her the sex of our baby. To prevent a fetus sex debacle, I said I would, by default, refer to our baby as He.

This plan didn't sit well. But I had made my case sufficiently enough for my wife to sympathize with me; we agreed we would ask the sex to be revealed to both of us at the next ultrasound.

I should have been a lawyer.

But as we shared our plan with other couples, it became clear the consensus was that this decision should be the woman's alone since she is the one who is pregnant; the one whose body is changing; the one who's experiencing morning sickness, etc. I felt this was the first of many examples of the father trying desperately to connect and yet being left on the sidelines due to circumstances beyond his control.

-"What names are you considering?" they would ask.

-"We haven't thought that far ahead," I would answer.

Wrong answer.

Your best bet is to plan in advance and have ready a boy's name and a girl's name, even if they are not the ones you plan to use when the baby is born. If you are armed and ready and can respond quickly with "Zanzibar, after my grandfather" or "Waikiki, after her Hawaiian grandmother," then you may only have to listen to a half-dozen or so suggestions from the person standing in front of you.

If you answer honestly: "We had not thought that far ahead," stand ready for a machine gun response, including possible names of living people, dead people, popular names, baby-naming websites, baby-naming books, popular actors names and what said actors are naming *their* babies. My polite smile-and-nod became so practiced, I might as well have been running a board meeting.

Of course, if you *do* cheat and make up a couple of names to throw to the wolves, be prepared for a different kind of disappointment, especially from the future grandparents. Honoring older, living relatives (and even *older* dead ones) through namesakes is a tradition the older generation will expect to be upheld. Since there are at least four grandparents to consider (each with parents of their own) and only *one* baby, this task is next to impossible. It is contrary to basic laws of the universe to be able to honor one family member while not insulting the others. Maybe that's one reason most religions see having children as such a blessing; after your 12th child, you've probably managed to satisfy everyone to the point they've actually started speaking to you again. I come from a Jewish family, so—although Christopher and Christian were always among my favorite boys names—there was no way it would be worth my while telling my parents my son's name begins with 'Christ.' It's just not worth it. Especially since longevity runs in our family; I'd be paying a steep emotional price for a very long time.

At least the dilemma of baby-naming is a stress born equally by both parents-to-be. "What are you going to name the baby?" is a question directed to the mother and the father. My wife was fielding just as many suggestions as I was.

Picking a name, however, was just about the last question asked equally of both of us; after that, the focus shifted dramatically towards the mother-to-be. It all starts with the question that would make a great drinking game: "How is she feeling?"

· SERENITY TIP FOR THE iDAD ·

Plug in. Have answers. Be interested—not for everyone else but as a reminder to your spouse that her husband is excited to be a dad.

BACK FROM THE FUTURE

From Blog to Books

Inspired by the MenGetPregnantToo.com Post: Yeah, I Know.
I Was Like That Too, Before Kids.
Published: July 17, 2011

Here is an interesting exercise for new parents: Each of you make a list of three things you *love* to do and stick it to the fridge. Once the baby comes, not only is there less of an *opportunity* to do those things, the *will* to do them also withers away. This is due purely to mathematics. Right now there are two adults, no children; therefore, you have a 50 percent chance of partaking in an activity of your choosing. Once you're involved in that activity, you only need share it or tailor the experience to one other person. With a baby, the number of humans in the household is increased by 50 percent. HOWEVER, this new human requires *exponentially* more attention and may participate in exponentially *fewer* activities. The newcomer will not be able to ride a rollercoaster for another six or seven years, and will not be able to sit through Shakespeare for at least another decade. This doesn't mean this new, little fun-sucker doesn't come with its own perks. Nor does it mean you can't make arrangements to hop on a rollercoaster or vacation in Stratford (do *not* see *The Winter's Tale* if you're a new parent...bad things happen to the baby, at least initially), but everything takes planning. Before you know it, a few years have gone by and you rediscover a pleasure that was such a distant memory, you had forgotten you ever enjoyed it in the first place. Before you know it, the only answer to "What's new?" becomes your latest tale of parenthood. From the blog:

> Caught a rebroadcast of Billy Joel's 2008 concert in New York City since they demolished Shea Stadium. Spectacular show. Made me wanna get a

grand piano. Made me wanna be a rock star. Made me notice how—at great rock shows—strangers never hesitate to smile at each other. Made me remember life before kids.

Now? Peter Gabriel's coming to town? Meh. I'm kinda tired, tickets are kinda pricey.

Wasn't the case when I was a D.I.N.K. (Double Income No Kids.) When I started dating my now-wife, we didn't want kids. We both worked odd hours, which often meant slow mornings with coffee, newspapers and morning *adult* television. Ya know, like, the news...or, like, "Good Morning America"...or, like, going back to bed after breakfast. We would also often work late, which meant bottles of wine being opened *after* midnight as opposed to bottles of formula being reheated at 3 a.m. It meant listening to full albums (yes, kids, artists used to release entire collections of songs, all at once) until the wee hours of the morning.

Ironically, I always liked children and always had a way with babies. I loved holding them, cooing at them, making them smile by digging my nose into their bellies. It's just that once I reached an age when I could have my own, I kinda went 'meh,' I'm kinda ok with it just being us. I'm likin' the lattes and last minute movies. I'm diggin' the urge to rent roller blades and then walk the whole way back 'cause my legs are kinda tired. And, you know what? On the way back, think I'm gonna grab myself an ice coffee.

Other people's children never bothered me either. Nor did some parents' tendencies to prattle on about nothing other than being a parent. I enjoyed their stories, and after all, once I talked about my latte and roller blades, I was pretty much done. Not everyone I knew was tolerant of baby stories, however. In one famous exchange, I witnessed a colleague of mine, who was single and spent nearly all his income on world travel, bark at another colleague concerning the frequency with which the latter would bring in pictures of his young son. The response was impeccable: "Buddy, when you stop bringing in your goddamn vacation photos, I'll stop bringing in baby pictures."

Parent 1, S.I.N.K. (Single Income No Kids) 0.

I still *do not* subscribe to the parenting mantra that gets regurgitated so often at the wrong times to the wrong people: "Children are a blessing. Without children, your life is just a little bit empty. It's something you don't understand unless you have kids."

Bullshit.

People who want kids should have kids. People who don't want kids should *not* have kids. As a matter of fact, some of the people who want kids should *not* have kids, and some of those who don't want 'em would probably make fantastic parents, if for no other reason than

their ability to think before they act. I can easily understand why a childless individual would find parents
monotonous. We *do* talk about our kids all the time. When
we're not comparing them to other kids, we're selling
checklists on street corners of their latest accomplish-
ments or cute moments. You know, not everybody cares.
But, you know, it's kinda like that person who is always
talking about work; it's not wrong, it's what they do for
eight hours a day. And when you take away from 24 hours
the eight hours during which you're asleep, plus the time
occupied with the mundane—groceries, showering, going
to the bathroom, sitting in traffic—most of what's left if
you're employed outside the home is work. Conversely,
when you are raising children, *that* is what you do with
most of your time, the rest of it is occupied with activities
much more banal.

We also always talk about our kids because we are
still, each day, discovering them for the first time. We're
also new at this, and it's a pretty big deal. My wife once
described being a parent as the most intense relationship
she's ever had. Talking about it is one way to shed the
nervous energy, the discovery of this developing spirit. It's
like the world becomes a psychiatrist for the person who is
now responsible for the education, emotional and physical wellness, intellectual development, clothing, nutrition
and eventual dating habits of another human being. And it
all starts with a blob of sleeplessness and excrement. We
don't want to bore you, but we can't help it. Just know that

we know we can be boring. We were D.I.N.K.s and chose to become otherwise. We fled Xanadu.

I realized, though, sitting on my couch watching Billy Joel rock Shae Stadium, that perhaps there is a difference between *becoming* a father and *turning* into one. I think I'm going to start pushing myself towards an odd event or two I used to enjoy as a D.I.N.K. but have since left behind. If you do the same, reader, perhaps we could be strangers smiling at each other from a couple of rows apart in a stadium somewhere. You'll know it's me; I'll be the guy who leaves before the encore—gotta get up with the baby tomorrow.

CHAPTER 7

How is She Feeling?

Ahhhh...sweet pregnancy. There is no feeling like waking up the morning after you've begun to spread The News. At first, while still groggy, you may ask yourself 'Something's new today. What is it?' And then you remember—my wife is pregnant *and everybody knows it!* For the next long while—especially in a family with so few grandchildren—you are the center of attention. Everyone will be buzzing; your parents will call two friends, who, in turn, will call two friends, who will call two friends, and before you know it, you are on the equivalent of the front cover of your life's *New York Times Magazine*. There could be no better start to the day...if it weren't for your wife not looking so well.

If you have ever taken the time to contemplate the human body and how it works, there is no denying it is a miracle of biblical proportions. Take something as simple as thirst: Your body—much like the planet itself—is composed largely of water. When the proportion of water-to-body-mass is even slightly off, your brain receives a message from your muscles, skin and organs that they need hydration. Your brain then takes over by transmitting a specific set of electrical impulses that your conscious mind interprets as thirst. This mechanism is something you are born with and it is with you until the day you die. Hydration is so important that one of the only real functions a human baby can perform autonomously at birth is drink. All of us are well acquainted with the body's other innate function: the disposal of waste. Once the body is properly hydrated, it sends any unneeded liquid into a holding area—the bladder—for disposal at its earliest convenience.

That is just a layman's short version of one of the body's most basic functions; not to mention other concrete examples such as hunger, temperature regulation and sleep. Some more abstract and fascinating ones are dreaming, desire, anger and all the other human emotions.

While the body is a miracle, it is also very delicate and very susceptible to even the smallest of changes. Dust in your nose? A sneeze. Dust in your lungs? A cough.

So imagine how a body is trying to cope with a newly fertilized egg—a growing human being—attached to the wall of a uterus. This new life requires a mother to keep it properly nourished and hydrated; her body temperature should be kept normal, and she needs to get enough exercise and enough rest while her body oversees the growth of fetus from microscopic organism to a seven-or-so-pound baby. The body has its own way of keeping a mother in check; morning sickness is one of them. It has a medical name: *emesis gravidarum* or N.V.P. It is also known by less clinical names such as throwing up and feeling really lousy—and believe me, those are two of the more polite words used to describe it. Doctors will tell you that while it is unpleasant, it is not dangerous. Tell that to husbands. They will also tell you that nausea and vomiting in the early stages of pregnancy can happen at any time of day, not just in the mornings.

There is no known cause, although the preponderance of evidence blames it on a hormonal imbalance—most likely caused by the human being growing inside you. Some of the over-the-counter treatments range from something one would find in a loot bag, to the kind of alternative treatments a cynical, nauseous pregnant woman might associate with voodoo. Treatments include the following:

"Preggie Pop": lollipops in flavors known to reduce nausea. (Available flavors include: ginger, mint, lavender, sour raspberry, sour lemon and sour tangerine.)

"Sea Bands": wristbands that use acupressure pulse points to fight nausea.

"Relief Band Device": a device that can be worn continuously for relief of mild to moderate nausea and vomiting associated with pregnancy,

And, finally, good old **"Vitamin B6":** Taking Vitamin B6 (50 mg) daily has been shown to help with pregnancy-induced nausea.[4]

Voilà, I have just saved you a three-hour wait in a doctor's office.

The symptoms can continue for months. It is also the first real post-conception test of a relationship, as well as the beginning of a debate that will continue until your children are in university or gainfully employed: How to look after others, while remembering to look after yourself.

A little history of my and my wife's relationship that will help you understand my arguments in this debate and may hopefully act as the voice for millions of men who are in a similar situation.

Before we were married, my wife lived in another city. She was working 10 hours a day in a very stressful job that had her

---

4   http://www.americanpregnancy.org/pregnancyhealth/survivingmorningsickness.html

squeezing in a coffee and a muffin during the 10 or so minutes she could get away from her desk. It was definitely NOT how she saw her future. A part-time position became available near me, so she quit her out of town job and we moved in together; the idea being she could look for full-time work after the move was over. Financially, it was very doable and, hey, love always wins.

Things were going so well, we married and decided we wanted to have children. We were in the unique position of me being employed full-time and her working permanent weekends. This would allow one of us to be home with our child right up until he or she would be school age; there would be no need for daycare.

All this is to say that once pregnancy was upon us, like so many other fathers-to-be, I was at work all day while my wife was becoming reacquainted with nausea and dizziness in a way she hadn't since parties in college.

Now throw in a touch of influenza.

To most of us, influenza is the proper name of a virus we normally call the flu. By and large, in healthy humans it causes fever, nausea, vomiting, diarrhea and fatigue over a period of several days or weeks. In extreme cases, it can be fatal. Doctors will tell you to drink a lot of clear liquids, eat healthy foods, get plenty of rest, perhaps increase your intake of vitamin C, perhaps include a dose of echinacea and avoid junk food, tobacco and alcohol.

Most of these things are already on the 'must do' list for a pregnant woman. In other words, when a husband phones an emergency healthcare number and says his pregnant wife has the flu, what can be done? The answer is this: Take two Tylenol and call me in the morning. Lucky me, getting to be the messenger.

Despite her ragged condition, my wife's pregnancy was giving me a new lift at work; I was boastful and proud. I, for the first time, instead of being bored listening to colleagues' parenting stories, was riveted. I couldn't wait to come home each day and check my wife's physical profile; was there a bump? Was the bump I was seeing real or imagined? This excitement was something I would try to subdue during my wife's battle with the first trimester, as much for her as for me. I was as concerned for her health and comfort as I was excited about her pregnancy. This being the first time for both of us, we were both impatiently wondering when we would see the end of these weeks of horrible symptoms, which were giving my wife the pallor of a passenger on SS *Minnow*.

And I could imagine that, from her flu-infested perspective, a husband who has been away all day in the world of the healthy and comes bounding through the door wanting to examine your silhouette, is about as welcome as trying to rid yourself of a headache by smashing your foot with a hammer. So the search for the proper balance began.

For many people marriage is really the first test for each party at being a primary caregiver. There tends to be no more (or at least, hopefully a lot less than there used to be) turning to your own Mummy and Daddy for care and support. You turn to each other first. Any experienced caregiver will tell you, one of the hardest lessons to learn is that there are times you have to put *yourself* first. It is a mantra often spoken between mothers, both during and after pregnancy. But putting themselves first is often what fathers, both during and after their wife's pregnancy, are criticized for. The truth is, we were never taught how to strike a balance.

§

"They mean well."

It's an expression I hate. It seems to be the go-to defense for anyone who has socially misstepped, wronged their family or their neighbor or their friend. "I did what I thought was best." Yes, but it was stupid, and you messed things up. Don't we all do what we think is best? Even the nastiest villains in movies and soap operas are always motivated by the fact they feel *someone* is benefitting from their malfeasance. Darth Vader was wonderfully loyal and devoted to the Dark Side.

I always hated that expression "They mean well," except as it pertains to expectant fathers. The absolute truth of all good husbands is that they are doing what they think is best within the parameters of their experience and emotions and cultural construction.

When we walk in the door and ask "How are you feeling?" for the 20th time, it is a question couching a different intention. Firstly, of course, we actually care to know how you are feeling. Secondly, the question is a thermometer to gauge the temperature of your mood. Anyone who has dated for more than a month knows that "I'm fine" can mean anything from "I'm fine" to "Screw you!" Often when a man asks "How are you feeling?" it can be translated directly to "Are you in a good mood?" because, quite frankly, men are flying blind. All the research, the self-help books and the talk shows cannot possibly permit a man to understand what a pregnant woman is feeling, especially where morning sickness is concerned. Damn that *emesis gravidarum.* We have had colds, flues and hangovers. The treatments were cold medicine, flu medicine, days off work and greasy food. Now, there is our partner, who is experiencing these symptoms brought on by *our* lifelong dream of becoming a parent, and she cannot take cold medicine or flu medicine, and she is trying desperately to save her sick and vacations days for when the baby comes. And if you offer her greasy food, hoping that—as with a hangover—it'll make things any better, prepare yourself for a Linda Blair demonstration.

The real irony in all this is there is no real support system for either the pregnant woman or for the father-to-be. In my experience, while sitting at work and listening to women talk about other women and their pregnancy symptoms, they are quite unforgiving. Half of those who have gone through it offer little support and are driven by the 'I went through it, so now so do you' militant philosophy. The other half experienced *no* adverse symptoms during their pregnancy, so they think there is fakery involved.

As far as men go, there is a similar division. Those without children stare right past you as you tell your stories. They're contemplating the spider on the wall behind your ear, hoping for the subject to change before the season does. The fathers in the room hear your feelings of helplessness as venting and sit anxiously like horses in the starting gate waiting to complain about *their* wives. The answer men give men to the statement "I wish there was something I could do about my wife's morning sickness" is "There is. Get out of the house."

While the pregnant, seasick mom battles her own voyage for the first trimester, the husband is dealing with his own mounting anxieties.

Aside from the general helplessness we feel at being... helpless, our world is changing, too. Before pregnancy, a man driving in life's car will look no farther than three or four blocks ahead. Suddenly, with a son or a daughter on the way, we become cursed with the need to peer as far as possible toward the horizon. Each paycheck is an examination of the rest of our lives: 'Is this forever?' 'Am I making enough money?' 'Is this the career I want for myself?' We are also, hopefully, being somewhat domesticated as a result of *emesis gravidarum*; even if we were doing our share before the pregnancy, Vomitus Maximus will naturally steer us to do a little more. While the baby is not physically growing within us, we are certainly being tweaked emotionally. One of the most difficult emotional situations a father-to-be has to deal with is this: To whom can we turn to openly discuss our nerves and angst?

§

While a woman's peers may not always be knocking on the door with bowls full of support for their pregnant friend, the couple's family do just the opposite. The outpouring of care and concern families show toward a pregnant woman can trigger very conflicting feelings within her husband. For the mother-to-be, phone calls and well wishes and offerings of soup and 'what worked for me' solutions are a huge relief. They are a blessed necessity. They provide a woman with comfort and the knowledge that, despite how lousy she feels, her family is there for her; as do the anecdotes from mothers and mothers-in-law who have experienced these wicked symptoms and remind her 'This, too, shall pass.'

The dad-to-be is in a different headspace; he's nervous, feeling both helpless at not having all the answers and downright useless after uttering the 40th 'I love you' and 'It'll be okay.' The dad also answers the phone and always fields the same first question:

-"How is she?"

-"She's tired, she's listless, she's nauseous, she's hungry but doesn't want to eat and she's wondering if she'll ever feel better. She's tired of eating crackers."

-"Okay, well, give her my love, and tell her to keep her chin up."

-"'K. Bye."

-"Bye."

...By-the-way, I'm not so hot, either, I would never get the chance to say. *I'm so excited and nervous about the baby, I didn't sleep last night. I wish there was more I could do, but the more I offer to help, the more I feel like I'm getting in the way. I want to offer her things without feeling she wishes I would stop offering her things. I would really like to talk to someone about this; someone who doesn't either have something better to do or respond with 'Yeah? Try pushing a cantaloupe out a mail slot.'*

Phone rings.

-"Hello?"

-"Hi! How is she?"

Any sensitive, logical man realizes what is happening. This is all a natural reaction to someone going through something extraordinary for the first time. Pregnancy is something everyone understands. There she is, she has a baby growing in her belly, and it's throwing things out of whack. This is no time for a non-pregnant husband to be whining about a lack of a psychological airbag. This is the time to shine, to step up, to show 'em what you're made of, etc. The alternative is to risk seeming selfish. BUT, and this is a big *BUT*, could this be the watershed period upon which future behavior is patterned? If a husband, during the nine months of a woman's pregnancy feels that this is not his time to talk about his fears and anxieties, how easy will it be to begin doing so in another nine months or 10 years down the road? One of the most popular complaints about men is that they don't open up, that they never share their feelings and that they're insensitive. One of the reasons for this is the type of sounding board that surrounds them. It is a Catch-22 that often has women telling their men to talk about their feelings. Yet when men are ready to say "What about my feelings?" it seems to come out at the wrong time. That is why iDADs sometimes approach talking about their emotions the same way one would go about jumping into a cold pool—you put your toe in first and see how inhospitable the water really is.

That being said, anyone who has jumped into a cool pool will tell you, it's not so bad once you're in. Sometimes it is best to skip the temperature test and just dive in headfirst.

Or you can take up jogging.

· SUPPORT TIP FOR THE iDAD ·

Put yourself first, even for an hour. Being temporarily selfish with your time will make being selfless later on much easier.

BACK FROM THE FUTURE

From Blog to Book

Inspired by the MenGetPregnantToo.com Post: Men, Aren't You Tired of Women Saying You Won't Open Up? Published: February 24, 2012

I eventually realized that, as much as women complain about men's lack of communication skills, they are not entirely unjustified. As I write about in this post, men don't do themselves any favors. Many of us simply won't share:

I mean, what's with that??

Granted there are many of us who won't (open up). For the sake of simplicity, let's refer to them (non-sharers) as *'They'* for the duration of this post.

They are plentiful. *They* have been the purveyors of the male stereotype for 10,000 years, give or take a Father's Day.

But, *They* have a soft underbelly; a secret kept hidden even from themselves. That secret is *Us*...

They may be like pit bulls, but *we* are that spot near their hindquarter that makes their paw flap when you scratch it.

When someone offers us a lollypop, we don't think of "suck this" jokes...we think of cavities.

When our shirt is wrinkled, not only do we insist on ironing it (ourselves!) before heading out the door, we pad the Sunbeam with a facecloth so it won't burn the fabric. Sure, we like ordering pizza, but you know what we *really* like? Making it from scratch, with quick-rise yeast and fresh basil and sun-dried tomatoes and Bocconcini cheese (which *doesn't* make us think of testicles).

On our Facebook pages, sure, we like "Spartacus" and "Dexter", but we also like the movie *Fame* (the original, not the remake) and *Saturday Night Fever* and *Dances with Wolves*...because we cry at the end...those poor Sioux. (Don't believe me? Check out my page.)

But my real point about fathers and daddies never being included in page headers is, it's time to gather as an online community and have a voice. Not as an isolated group of metrosexuals but a blend of women and men, mothers and fathers, Cro-Magnons and...*Me*...*Us*...*We*. It's not about finding a platform on which we can separate ourselves from others; it's about giving opportunities for contrarians to share points of view. Dads, join the mommy groups. Moms, join the daddy groups. (Hang on, I've got to go start one with all my free time.)

I'll bet you all a *Beaches* movie night you'll be surprised at the quantity of common ground. At the very least *We* can defend ourselves to *Them,* and *They* to *Us.*

Until then, I'll continue to sign up on pages with pink backgrounds and perfume giveaways and to file my posts under "mommies and babies" because I certainly am more welcome there than at "pregnant and breastfeeding."

And, by the way...*We* do have nachos and beer during the Super Bowl while watching these behemoths smash into each other...22 men in tights heaped in a pile. (Yeah, like *We're* the ones with the problem.)

Gotta go...my weekly recipe just popped into my inbox.

CHAPTER 8

Kenny, This is Your Life Calling

˅ **PET PEEVE OF THE iDAD** ˅

Suggestions from people on how to fix the barn door
after the cows have come home.

E veryone has an opinion about *everything* related to your baby: the name, for instance.

But, before a name could be chosen, the sex was to be determined. Everyone has an opinion about this, as well. Everyone assumes the man wants a boy to play football with; to play hockey with; to have a beer with; to grunt with and to smell bad with. Of course, everyone knows that for your first baby there is only one correct answer when asked about the sex of a baby: "I don't care, as long as it's healthy." This is true, for the most part. In my experience this is one of those irrational fears: admitting to someone that you may have a preference for either a boy or a girl. Of course, given the choice of an unhealthy baby or a healthy one of random sex, everyone would chose a child's health over a specific sex. The question itself is unfair. It's like asking me: Would you rather go to Hawaii during a hurricane or stay home? Of course, I would stay home if the alternative was dodging debris in Maui. This doesn't mean that during the average Canadian winter I would prefer to be at home than be in Hawaii.

My preference was for a girl. Why? Because I *was* a boy; I know what boys were like when I was growing up. I know what *I* was like growing up. I felt boys were very physically competitive; a trait I did not share. When I was young, I always felt more comfortable with girls than boys. Not much has changed growing up; I feel more relaxed around women than I do men. I still find men can be very competitive and less open to discussing life's issues, often hiding behind them with sarcasm...and beer. I know women say girls can be just as evil. They tease and torment; their torture is more emotional and less physical, thereby making it more damaging. Women can be catty and competitive, as well. But I didn't grow up a girl, and I am not a woman. My preference is based on my experience. This is not to say that my son will necessarily have all—or even any—of the less desirable traits I witnessed in my male friends growing up, but if someone were to ask me if I preferred a little boy or a little girl, I would answer honestly.

Of course, everyone has opinions pertaining to which sex is easier. Boys are supposedly easier as teens but more difficult as toddlers. Girls are said to be easier babies, but miserable teenagers. Everyone has an answer. I remember doing some pretty horrible things as a teenager. I also remember my sister as a teen saying things to my mother that a wrestler wouldn't say to the guy he had on the ropes. But I wouldn't mind if my son were like me, or if my daughter were like my sister; we survived quite nicely, sometimes despite ourselves and our surroundings.

§

Back at the hospital for the ultrasound. Today is the day we will find out the sex of this little critter. After today, it will no longer be 'It.' 'It' will be 'He' or 'She.' We had been in the waiting room for a while, listening for our names to be called, and after two cups of hospital coffee, I went to find the men's room. Being the investigative genius that I am, I followed the conspicuous sign on the wall that read "Washroom," with an arrow next to it pointing down the hall. Following the arrow, I came across a women's washroom. Knowing our healthcare system the way I do, I knew I had more than enough time to search for the men's room before we were called in for the exam. I covered a lot of ground in all directions during my search for the men's room, and in my travels, passed by two other women's bathrooms. Asking a nurse or doctor where the bathroom was would make me feel a little like Coco the monkey, but when you gotta go, you gotta go, right? Who would understand that better than the staff in an obstetrics ward?

-"Excuse me, where are the washrooms?"

-"Second floor, down the stairs on your left."

-"Really? There are no men's rooms on this floor?"

-"No, sir. It's an obstetrics floor in the Women's Pavilion."

Off you go, Coco.

I could imagine the escalation were I to ask her if she was aware that men are 50 percent responsible for the existence of a maternity ward. Not to mention the literature in the waiting room promoting the father's complete participation in the birthing process. Apparently, participating in fatherhood is much like a night at the opera; it's a beautiful thing, but you should go to the washroom before you leave the house.

Relieved, and...*relieved* after returning to the Women's Pavilion, I reported with my wife to the exam room. Being next to her while she was being prepared for an ultrasound also made me feel a little like Coco (again, the Monkey, not Chanel). I am seated on my little stool, listening patiently as the technician prepares my wife for the procedure. All the instructions and questions are directed towards the pregnant lady, as they should be. But there are constantly these moments of awkwardness: My stool is in the way of the machine. 'Please move over there, sir.' I would like to hold her hand, but there is nowhere to put our jackets, so, much like accompanying her to a ladies clothing store, I'm doubling as a coat rack. But I have a silly smile on my face, anyway, because I'm thrilled at being here to discover the sex of the baby; this is simply a great way to spend an afternoon. The scan begins. The time it's taking for the technician to get around to revealing whether I'm to have a son or daughter seems painfully long. First, all the measurements must be taken to be sure the baby's growth is following the proper curve. Measure the head, measure the neck, check the heart. Eventually she asks the question:

-"Would you like to know the sex of the baby?"

-"Yes." I would also like a men's washroom installed on this floor, but I assume that is a separate department.

The paddle moves down along my wife's belly. The image on the monitor changes along with the movement of the paddle. I'm amazed at the utilitarian touch the technician has, pushing and prodding in different directions like someone using a metal detector on a comforter. Finally, we get a clear shot. Suddenly, the image on the screen is a baby viewed from the bottom up; a grainy black and white image, much like an x-ray plus body tissue. The angle is as though the scan is taken of a baby sitting on a toilet, but the camera is in the toilet pointing upwards. We could clearly see the back of two little thighs joining at a little rump, and in between the thighs—tiny testicles and an even tinier penis.

-"It's a boy," she says.

There is a moment of quiet emotion. It's funny and strange the way the body produces tears during moments of both joy and sadness. This was certainly one of joy. Not joy at finding out that it is a boy or that it's healthy. It is the feeling of reassurance and validation that this is really happening. As much as there are several-times-daily discussions with friends, colleagues and family members about the baby, and as much as you spend your days reading websites and magazines trying to get a clearer picture of what's in store for a new parent, there is nothing like a physical image and a clean medical bill of health to validate your future as a parent. It was a sense of exhilaration and accomplishment I had never experienced before. I couldn't wait to meet my son.

§

After the elation of the ultrasound, the bounce was soon to be taken out of my step. We moved to a smaller room to meet with the obstetrics nurse. She began going through a series of routine questions about my wife's health, diet, general physical state, sleep pattern and energy level. She also asked my wife for a urine sample and took some blood.

After the testing was complete, she went through the history of the file.

-"I see you are Rh negative," she said to my wife.

-"Yes, they told me that last time I was here."

-"Did they explain to you what that means?"

Both of us admitted we had received an explanation, but that now, a couple of months later, we couldn't explain clearly what that was. Rh, she explained, is a protein produced in the blood. Since my wife lacks this protein, there is a risk to the baby should the baby's father be Rh *positive*. The good news is, the problem is easily solved by giving my wife a couple of injections at certain points during the pregnancy. I asked what I thought was a rather obvious question:

-"If the risk to the fetus is only a result of the father being Rh *positive*, why not simply give me a blood test? Maybe the injections won't be necessary."

The nurse's response was coldly logical:

-"Because we can never assume that the husband is the baby's father."

Silence.

Were I a Vulcan, I would have felt no emotion whatsoever. It made perfect sense; half of all marriages end in divorce, which means there is probably a fair bit if infidelity out there. When you have a couple in front of you expecting a baby, what woman would choose that moment to reveal to the nurse, and to her husband, that she had had an affair and the baby might belong to another man? The injections made sense. Please proceed, thank you. I would never believe for a moment that my wife had had an extramarital affair. Still, it was like being hit in the back of the head with a softball while looking at a piece of art. There was no choice but to see the humor of the moment. Despite that, I couldn't help but wonder how a woman's feelings would be affected were the roles reversed. Imagine a woman, sitting next to a pregnant man and being told:

-"We can never assume the wife was faithful."

I think that if those roles were reversed, and the wife was having her devotion questioned by the obstetrics nurse, there would be many more arguments in the car on the way home.

The ride home was an exciting trip towards the next phase of the pregnancy and the final choosing of a name.

We had made a short list. We were looking at naming Him (as He could now be known) after grandparents, but attractive name choices were slim where my grandfathers were concerned: Moe or Harry (although Harry also had a nickname: Butch). We had narrowed the list down once we noticed there were several grandparents and family members on both sides whose names started with M. Another factor in picking the names was our respective nationalities and religions. My wife's background is Irish, English and Scottish Protestant; my side was Eastern European Jew. All this, coupled with the obvious factor of choosing a name that pleased both my wife and me, led us to agree on Mirren Oz.

Saint Mirren was the patron saint of the town of Paisley (as well as the patron saint of soccer—I wasn't a fan of European football, but I found it interesting the sport *had* a patron saint in the first place), and Oz is a Hebrew word meaning 'strong.'

Of course, once again there was no shortage of opinions from the gallery and even less hesitation to make themselves heard; my father for instance:

-"Why didn't you pick a Jewish name?"

-"We did. Oz is Hebrew."

-"Hebrew doesn't mean Jewish, and the way you pronounce it isn't the Jewish pronunciation; it's English."

Oy.

Also, through tears, my mother chimed in:

-"I was hoping you would name him after my father."

-"Mom, I did not want to name my son Moe."

-"What about Moses?"

-"What *about* Moses?!"

Back and forth it went, everyone expressing support or dismay or surprise or confusion. Why does having a baby also seem like an election call for everyone to register a vote about everything? As if it is not enough dealing with the unavoidable stresses and struggles—both physical and mental—that accompany you on a journey towards first-time parenthood, you have to appeal to the masses. You try your best not to fail your midterms. Occasionally, tempers boil over and you are forced to bite back:

-"You know why not Moses?! Because I don't *like* the name Moses. I know Moses is a great biblical figure; he's also a Hall of Fame basketball player. But it is *my* job to choose a name for *my* son that pleases *me* and my wife. How can there be an argument about choosing a name for *our* baby? Don't you think becoming a first-time parent is stressful enough?"

Then comes one of the more ironic answers your parents will ever give you:

-"Of course, I *know* it's stressful; I had *you* didn't I?"

And they wonder why you keep things from them, like the possibility of a genetic defect in the fetus or even the fact theat-she's pregnant in the first place. Sometimes, sharing information is just too much work.

This is the irony of this one experience that you absolutely, undeniably share with your parents: parenthood. Despite having gone through the same trials and decisions, they *still* second guess the most mundane details, a lot of sweating the small stuff. I understand concerns expressed from friends and especially parents when they are related to the child's health: Make sure she's getting enough rest. Make sure she's getting enough exercise, etc. They all want what's best for their friend, their son, their daughter and especially their first grandson. But the frills—the name, how much sex I *did* have, *am* having, and *will* have—those things are my business. Sometimes when the phone rings and the conversation begins, "Kenny, I was thinking a little more about the name, and I have a suggestion before it's too late…," I'm tempted to lie and say I recently had call waiting installed to handle all the telephone traffic: "Sorry I have to let you go. There's someone on the other line. My life is calling."

· SURVIVAL TIP FOR THE iDAD ·
Sometimes, when "No" doesn't work, stalling for nine months with "I'll think about it, thanks" works just fine.

CHAPTER 9

Self-Help, or How to Go Crazy Before Bedtime

˙ **PET PEEVE OF THE iDAD** ˙

All the experts with all the answers to all the questions
can't seem to agree with each other.

S ince my friends—be they single or married, with or without children—do not seem to provide me with the sort of 'help-line' advice I'm looking for, it behooves this father-to-be to seek expert advice elsewhere: in books, for instance. A quick Googling of "parenting books" turns up 1,180,000 hits. That's 1.18 *million*. That number drops to 5,000 when you search for "fathering books." Many of those are biographical, not mental-health related, or they're offering to teach you a certain specific skill set: building a baby room from scratch, for instance. Many books are written by comedians, actors and sports figures, with touching, first-person accounts of their lives with *their* fathers and how their dads influenced them. Most of the stories are remarkable, whether due to their humor or to their honest despair at a life nearly derailed by an abusive dad. Very few of these books help new fathers really prepare for fatherhood. There is an important distinction to be made: While there are few books serving as emotional guidelines for fathers-to-be in terms of emotional strength and how to build confidence as a dad before becoming a dad, there are *many* books helping men become better caregivers and support networks for their wives.

There are chapters on the importance of being a good listener; the importance of foot rubs and back rubs; and chapters on how to prepare a suitcase for the hospital. I especially love the chapters with a tone implying they are talking to a 6-year-old as it explains that a woman's water breaking is nothing to be afraid of; it is only natural; it is merely a sign that the baby is on its way and you are now mere hours from becoming a daddy. Thank you for helping me to determine the difference between amniotic fluid and Soylent Green. Of course, all chapters end with a similar sentiment: 'Above all, try to keep calm, as this will help you and your wife as you reassure her and keep her comfortable.' Fair enough. Where are the chapters on dealing with in-laws, on finding your own source of reassurance and those discussing the importance of a father's role in the pregnancy (other than keeping everyone comfortable)? There are no books that point out that a father is also looking for reassurance, and the guy in the corner is not just a 'nervous dad-in-waiting,' he is the other half of a pregnant couple.

Despite feeling neglected, I felt it was my duty to read what was available, if for no other reason than to have some conversation to contribute—other than a grunt—as my wife poured over *her* literature. It did not take long before I felt lost among the thousands of pages of advice and opinions. The varieties of contradictory hypotheses were bewildering. The information highway has found its own enemy: itself. The potential wealth of information available in the guru industry is surpassed only by the hunger and quest by the public for more gurus. There is a voice out there to support any point of view; they all offer different answers to the same questions: What is normal? What is not? And who can really define normal, anyway? There is a similar rhythm to the advice: Book 'A' stipulates you should definitely follow a specific course of action; book 'B' stipulates you should definitely *not* follow that same course of action, and somewhere toward the end of books 'A' and 'B,' they will both stipulate that above all, you should do what makes you happy.

Among the most popular books, especially for men, are the 'what is happening to the fetus this week' series. These are of interest to husbands because it is their connection to the baby growing within someone else. My wife is a healthy person, so there is redundancy in me telling her that according to a certain pregnancy manual, she should be eating healthy foods, keeping up some moderate exercise and staying away from cigarettes and alcohol (although—especially where alcohol is concerned—there is some debate; I'll let you chase the M.D.s for the answers).

I became truly fascinated with the week-to-week development of my son. One week he grows a fingernail. One week he grows a toe, then an ear, then some hair. One week he sucks his thumb. By now he has quadrupled in size since the date of conception. Amazing.

Of course, the more one reads about something the size of a thumb growing within your wife's belly, the more one tends to worry about the fragility of something merely the size of a thumb growing within your wife's belly. While I would fall into bed at the end of the day exhausted from the combination of office work and adrenaline and excitement about the baby, the thoughts of the possible peril facing that little, gestating snow pea would inevitably leave me awake, staring at the ceiling. Of course, I'm a rational guy; the earth has a population of 7 billion people, a large portion of whom have already given, or will one day, give birth. For tens of thousands of years women have been giving birth under much less favorable conditions than exist today: under trees, on rocks, on beaches, in caves, in jungles, surrounded by lions and tigers and bears (oh, my)! I was pretty sure that a healthy woman, in a queen size bed in the suburbs, had a fairly good chance of a normal pregnancy and delivery. But in these books there is such emphasis on the delicate balance of rest and nutrition required to make sure nothing goes wrong that there are a lot of 'buts' in these books. Such-and-such should be fine, *but* it's not ideal. Jogging, walking up and down flights of stairs and dancing were all on various 'do' *and* 'don't' lists. I mean, how can that little lima bean manage to hang on while mom is *jogging*?

I tried not to think about it and to get some sleep, but tomorrow, when I'm standing farther than thirty feet away from people smoking, do I run over and ask them to stop?...*Stop thinking about it and get to sleep!* The mantra was always the same: It'll be fine.

My inner voice was my own worst enemy. I found it difficult to assemble a group of men with whom I could banter about all these worries. Women have a network of experienced mothers to turn to. Try to get a group of men together to discuss an unborn fetus; you might as well tell them you're organizing a weekly cross-stitching class.

I learned to trust my instincts. I found a book or two that made sense to me, books that I felt dealt with pregnancy in a reasonable way and spoke to me in a non-condescending tone. I took the information from those books that I felt was useful. As for the rest of them? During hot, sleepless nights worrying about my abilities to parent, they did a fine job of propping up the window-unit air conditioner.

· SELF-HELP TIP FOR THE iDAD ·
Information and suggestion are the experts' responsibilities; interpretation is yours. Read with a healthy filter.

CHAPTER *10*

Hands-Off My Diet! — Where Father-hood and a Woman's Body Collide

I don't smoke. I don't drink excessively. (Why is *not* drinking always followed by a qualifier by people like me?)

But, I am a potato chip addict.

It's true, according to at least one definition of 'addicted':

The repeated use of a substance or behavior despite clear evidence of negative consequences resulting from the use of the substance or behavior. Addiction usually has two components – physical addiction and psychological addiction.

Even the healthiest potato chip is very high in salt and low in most vitamins, minerals and nutrients. They also leave me feeling a general malaise the morning after eating a bag of them. (I don't mean one of those cute bags you give out during Halloween or even his bigger brother that hides in vending machines; I sit down with those 200g guys, the ones everyone else empties into a bowl to share with their friends during Super Bowl weekend). I wake up with a funny taste in my mouth and salt-induced swelling just about everywhere—a serious case of water-retention. Not to mention all the calories that are now lying unburned in my body, just waiting to transform themselves into love handles and a daddy gut.

Despite that, if I walk by a convenience store, I stand there talking to myself like a man delivering a knockout punch in a presidential debate, desperate to convince myself that I should keep walking…that I don't need them…they're not good for me…they're replacing the otherwise nutritious food I should be eating. Then I think about how *good* they are, about how much

I will enjoy sitting on the couch watching a movie with a cold beer and a bag of chips. I imagine eating them slowly, one by one at first, that large intact chip easily grabbed at the top of the bag, crunching, salty, vinegary, barbecuey, pickley, ketchupy... one chip at a time. Then, by the time I reach the middle of the bag, the chip—either due to the size of the potato, or breakage during transport—diminishes in size. I will therefore eat two at a time, then three, until, as I reach the bottom of the bag, I'm shoving handfuls of shards and scraps down my throat until there is nothing left. Then I will create a funnel along the side of the bag, smoothing it so any crumbs can slide unencumbered into my mouth. Then I put my lips to the edge of the bag and tip the whole thing over. Sad, really.

Finally, I will sit back, digest and look forward to my next bag of chips.

On a good week, I can easily consume four large bags.

My loving wife has never said a word about it. I'm an adult and she treats me like one; it's my body and she'll love me whether I look like David Hasselhoff or Dom Deluise. Vise-versa. Her body is her castle, and other than debates about her smoking (which she had already given up) we live and let live.

But NOW she's pregnant....(Insert macabre theme song and maniacal laugh here.)

Let the furious debate begin.

§

What a woman eats and how she takes care of herself when pregnant is a prime example of situations that put men on an emotional tightrope. It is the perfect storm of no-win situations.

"The baby is as much yours as it is mine" is a phrase spoken so often by mothers married to 'football' fathers: men who unplug from the dirty work of diapers and mealtime, but take over once Junior is old enough to toss a ball or go the movies. However, when a dad decides to plug in, how early is too early? Does a lack of physical attachment by definition mean less of an entitlement to an opinion about lifestyle choices that may affect the health of the fetus? After all, the baby's health is going to be of equal concern and responsibility to both the mother and the father. Why shouldn't that concern and responsibility begin during gestation?

One reason may be that when you are already experiencing morning sickness, weight gain and general malaise, the last thing an expectant mother needs is backseat health advice. Conversely, one of the few tools men have at their disposal during their partner's pregnancy is information. Reading books—especially the ones being read by your expectant spouse—is a great way to not only *show* your support but actually *be* supportive. Books written for expectant mothers are a wonderful tool for men, if for no other reason than when your wife begins a sentence with "the book says," she has a real sounding board—someone who has taken an interest in the literature and can either support its point of view or present a different interpretation based on the same information.

Much of this advice, however, is nutritional and health related; diet and exercise are among the most popular and divisive topics covered in pregnancy self-help literature. Some of these points of view are quite powerful and leave no room for discussion, such as this statement released by the U.S. Surgeon General in 2005:

> *U.S. Surgeon General Richard H. Carmona today warned pregnant women and women who may become pregnant to abstain from alcohol consumption in order to eliminate the chance of giving birth to a baby with any of the harmful effects of the Fetal Alcohol Spectrum Disorders (FASD). FASD is the full spectrum of birth defects caused by prenatal alcohol exposure.*[5]

Most research supports the complete abstinence from alcohol by women who are—or intend to become—pregnant.

So, here I am. The guy.

My wife has pulled through a tumultuous first trimester, full of side effects that would make a night on the *Poseidon* feel like an hour in a sensory deprivation tank. She is finally feeling like herself and we can now confirm our presence at social functions without the caveat: "We'll have to let you know how she's feeling."

We feel like a million bucks, sitting around a dinner table with a gaggle of our closest friends. We've finally both been sleeping well and it seems her pregnancy has shifted itself into cruise control; it looks like the worst of pregnant life is behind us. Surely, a little celebration is in order.

Then the host asks my wife the question:

-"Would you like a glass of wine?"

The response around the table, especially if the group is restricted to peers of our generation, is generally the same: tacit support for anything that will allow a pregnant woman to

---

5   http://www.surgeongeneral.gov/pressreleases/sg02222005.html

stretch her legs a little. Generally, the pregnant woman scans the group with an expression that betrays a delicate mix of guilt and exhilaration, and she inevitably permits herself the indulgence of a delicious glass of fruity, robust, aromatic red wine.

Who can blame her?

I'm sitting across the table; the forces of good and evil are doing battle at the speed of light in my head. We've all experienced this strange duality that exists seemingly for the sole purpose of separating mind, mouth and judgment.

My mind: It is analyzing all the data it has absorbed over the past few months during its study of the pregnant female and is searching frantically for the index card containing the information regarding alcohol consumption. The search results are clear and they draw a coldly logical conclusion: *Most research supports the complete abstinence from alcohol by women who are, or intend to become, pregnant.*

A millisecond has passed since the glass of wine has been offered.

My mental index card has sent my logical brain the information it requested, which is now booted to the next compartment: judgment.

I'm at a cerebral fork in the road.

Scenario 1: I suggest openly to my wife in front of a dinner table full of guests that perhaps a glass of wine is not the healthiest choice for our unborn son. Logically, it is certainly justifiable; the glass of alcohol itself is several times larger than the unborn child, and at 13 percent alcohol it will, at best, be of no benefit and may even do some harm to the baby, right? After all, I'm the husband...the dad...half of 'the parents.' If I believe something to be true and am supported by data, why should I not speak up?

Because we, around this table, are human beings with feelings, however flawed, passionate, and reactionary. Also because mental health, relaxation, social interaction, the benefits of celebration and the joy of the moment are all factors in the equation.

The situation is more than the sum of its parts.

Scenario 2: I say nothing. My wife will look at me and I'll give her a loving smile coupled with properly enthusiastic words of encouragement from the marriage playbook: "My goodness, honey, if there is *anyone* around this table who deserves a glass of wine, it's you. It's only once in a while, and most people know that an occasional glass of wine will do no harm. Heck, have one for me, too. I'll drive home."

She will enjoy her glass after giving me a kiss in acknowledgement of my selfless support. So why not just shut up and be encouraging? After all, I'm not the one who's had to deal with a trimester of misery.

Because I am a human being with feelings, however flawed, passionate, and reactionary.

Because my face will betray me, as will my mood, which will be changed ever so slightly by the tension in my gut.

Because I will spend the evening wondering if the glass or two of wine, on occasion, will even minutely affect the chances of having a perfectly healthy baby.

Because, at times, I can be a little particular and difficult.

And because I care.

Scale and grandeur aside, wars on battlefields have nothing on wars between making a judgment and choosing whether to verbalize it. How do we exercise enough self-control to say the right thing, though we may be thinking something very wrong?

Several full seconds have passed since my wife was offered the drink and I win the battle against my own poor judgment.

I opt for an upgraded Scenario 2. Or Scenario 2.1, if you will: I realize how well my wife knows me.

I tell her, of course, I think she should relax and have a drink and take a load off. A drink or two won't hurt.

I knew how badly she wanted that release. Not because of some sort of dependency or escapism but because months of discipline can take their toll; endless reading and digesting of advice on what to eat and drink, how much to exercise, the importance of sleep and relaxation in a world that does not easily permit relaxing, is in and of itself, exhausting.

This glass or two of indulgence is a shred of inclusion; a reminder that those things you enjoy most are not automatically and forever out of reach because of parenthood.

My support, though, was tempered with a reticence detectable only to the person at the table who has spent years knowing me as well as anyone could.

She knew.

She knew that my okay was laced with an 'I'm not sure,' as well as a dash of 'Do you think that's a good idea?'

To her credit, she understood and said nothing. The glass of wine was enjoyed by my wife drop by drop. Each sip held within it the politics of marriage, motherhood, pregnancy and love.

The question is, though: What if I had a stronger objection?

There are three points of view concerning drinking while pregnant: don't, do, and in moderation.

There are two opinions to be counted concerning drinking while pregnant: the mother's, and the father's.

What if the father *does* have a strong objection to the mother having a drink with dinner? Imagine the atmosphere created when an expectant mother is offered a drink and the expectant father says: "I don't think that's such a good idea."

From uptight and killjoy, to controlling and abusive, the adjectives would line up.

Perhaps this is an exaggeration, perhaps not. But domain over the health of the unborn child and a woman's control over her own body are concepts that can be so grey and nebulous to a father-to-be that the challenge to distinguish between them can be stressful.

Even as I write this, I want to tell myself to relax; it is not that big a deal. 'Back in the day' that may have been true. But this isn't 'the day'; this is now. There is much more information available to parents today, and though the literature is still tailored to women, men are now expected to try and keep up. We are told ignorance is no longer an option. Laundry, cooking, cleaning, diapers, hugging and kissing; these are things that are, and should be, mandatory for dads. However, we are still kept on the bench for the early innings of the game. The concept of 50/50 doesn't start during pregnancy; it starts at birth.

This is one of the reasons I discovered de-alcoholized beer. I enjoy a cold beer or two at the end of the day. Do I want to sit next to someone who is obliged to limit her enjoyment of wine and the occasional cold beer, only to subject her to the 'fitz' of a cap being twisted off a cool one, followed by the 'gulp... ahhh' of the golden brew slithering down my throat? No. Not nice. Tempting, in a sadistic sort of way, but not nice. Beer with 0.5 percent alcohol was a nice compromise. Sure it tastes like carbonated apple juice gone wrong, but anything for my sweetie. I actually grew accustomed to the stuff quite quickly. The irony of my choosing a beverage that I could share without hesitation with my pregnant wife is that she was so put off by the taste, she was rarely interested. Although, 0.5 percent mixed with ginger beer makes a great shandy and a nice summer treat for someone cutting back on sangria.

Alcohol is even more benign than cigarettes, though smokers disagree. They often compare tobacco addictions to heavy or even casual drinking. The argument is often made: "What harm is there in having a cigarette when Joe Blow drinks himself under the table three times a week at the local tavern and then hauls his inebriation home to his family?"

The only difference is, unlike second-hand smoke, Joe doesn't force the people around him to take a half-a-sip of booze for every one of his.

My point is this: The pregnancy and alcohol scenario becomes even more pressing where second-hand smoke is concerned. Restaurants and coffee shops were the real hot zones. Why? Because, *boy,* we love our coffee, my wife and I. I mean we are *real* coffee snobs: Arabica, Jamaican Blue Mountain, dark roast, medium roast. Should grounds be kept in the freezer or in a vacuum-sealed container or in a vacuum-sealed container *in* the freezer? We were serious about our coffee, as well as the ceremony surrounding the drinking of it. Drinking coffee and going somewhere together to sit and drink coffee became one of those rituals that did not exist for either of us before we were *us*. This little tropical bean, which when crushed and drained of its essence by hot water, becomes an elixir. It was a corner post of our weekly rituals. Of course, decaf took some getting used to.

What goes wonderfully with a hot coffee? Cigarettes. Jim Jarmusch named a movie after these partners. Within the past couple of years, more and more municipalities have passed blanket no-smoking laws, but this is not the case everywhere, and during my wife's pregnancy, it was not the case *anywhere*.

So here we are, walking into a coffee shop, desperate to get out of the house: her, enjoying a break from nausea and baby-talk; I, enjoying a break from her nausea and our baby-talk. We were both just looking to lose ourselves in a cup of Joe.

But there's this guy in the corner sucking on a Camel while sipping on a cappuccino. He seems really relaxed. If I took a drag on his Camel, I would look like E.T., but the atmosphere around this guy was one of such pure relaxation and contentment, that under most circumstances I would have been very tempted to join him. But standing next to my pregnant wife, I felt that tension building within me. I felt my blood pressure rise. I became agitated and very aware that this guy was making me desperate to get my wife out of this coffee shop. He was on the other side of a *very* large room. I couldn't smell the smoke; I couldn't even see any of it anywhere in our half of the restaurant. The experience became immediately unpleasant for me since I instantly began fighting my instinct to suggest to my wife that we run from this inferno. Fortunately, she, too, was bothered by the presence of second-hand smoke and suggested that we get our java to go. The decision was taken out of my hands. But my autonomic response was similar when faced with any of the common 'vices': smoke, alcohol, junk food, etc. How in control was I in any given situation? When does care become interpreted as obsession? At what point does the information obtained in self-help books concerning a healthy fetus begin to make you feel helpless?

I am lucky. I feel quite comfortable expressing my concerns about the baby's external environment. I have learned, however, that it is best for me to express these fears when we are removed from the situation, not just so the moment isn't ruined, but because I know I express myself better when I'm not being influenced by the stress of the situation. Also, for all things if there is one truth that I hold dear, even for the health of the fetus, it's 'everything in moderation.' One glass of wine or a chocolate bar can induce moments of pure joy, which can sometimes be few and far between during a pregnancy. I have to ask myself: Do I want to become an added source of stress for my wife in the name of protecting our child? No, because the stress itself is of no help to the baby or our marriage.

However, communication is vital. All those stores with all those shelves, holding all those books, are trying to do one thing: communicate. Why are they so popular? One reason is that couples, after a time, no longer take each other at face value. Sometimes a statement coming from a third party holds more value than one coming from your husband or wife, especially where health and medicine are concerned. That's why we love our books so much; they provide us with validity. How many times have you, while reading a self-help book, found a particular passage to be an ally and then read it aloud to your partner? It is a very diplomatic way of saying "I told you so."

These books are becoming the courtrooms of private opinion. There is nothing wrong with that. You'll soon discover there is an expert out there supporting each of us. Once again: Everything in moderation. Men: When something is important enough to you, use pillow time—with the self-help literature close-by on the nightstand—to express yourself.

And wives. If your husband is curled up next to you in bed, with a self-help book on his lap after he spent the day freaking out at you about such things as coffee and wine, consider yourselves lucky…it's as pregnant as he can be.

ˑ SELF-HELP TIP FOR THE iDAD ˑ
Before weighing in, ask yourself: "In 18 years, will this stress over a glass of wine have made a difference?"

Back From the Future

From Blog to Book

Inspired by the MenGetPregnantToo.com Post: Exercise?!
The Last Thing I Jogged Was My Memory.
Published: August 18, 2012

A word about bodies and health and image: During pregnancy, and for a while afterward, any household's focus on physicality is almost exclusively female-centric. Of course it is; her health and body, the baby's health and (especially) her feeling about each of these is greatly magnified. This focus continues after birth, as well as when a couple dozen pounds are shed. This leaves the mother pretty much on her own to regain the physical state she had known throughout her life up until this point.

As the baby grows up, however, a father can easily fall into similar parent traps. Time to work out is harder to find, as is time to relax. It is the latter that many fathers—such as myself—will gravitate to. Before long, we wonder where our energy went, just as I wondered in this post:

I have a stringent running schedule. It's like clockwork. It's a little OCD, really.

For about seven consecutive months I run three to four times a week. I'll work towards a half-marathon, one either in my hometown or a short drive away in Ottawa.

After the race, I'll intend to take a week off and begin training for a full marathon, imagining myself an uber-fit 40-year-old smoking all the 20-somethings who run races thinking they know what it means to be in shape.

But, inevitably, after the race weekend something important comes up, like a once-in-a-parent-of-young-children's-lifetime dinner and a movie with my wife. I'll skip running that evening. (I *never* run in the morning. I know there are parents of youngsters who wake even *earlier* than their kids to work out. Those parents are just plain crazy.)

The morning following Date Night (which is really just sitting next to each other in bucket seats rather than on the sofa, and watching a really big silver screen instead of the TV in the den) I'll sleep in and have a slow breakfast. I justify *that* laziness as an extension of Date Night.

A couple of days later I'll skip running because it's too hot. I'll skip the one after that because of some sort of appointment and the one after that because I haven't blogged frequently enough due to my rigorous training.

Then I'll take seven months off because I'm discouraged and out of shape.

So it goes: seven months on, seven off.

I'm at the tail end of the seven months off, and I'm feeling it. My back is stiff after watching "The Newsroom" back-to-back to "True Blood." My shoulder hurts when I lift one of my kids (Remember when you used to lift both of them simultaneously? Are they bigger, or are you older? The answer is 'yes.') Every 20 minutes or so, I flex my neck muscles and turn my head—the move is followed by a satisfying cracking noise where my head meets my body.

I need to get back out there. But, boy, I really don't want to.

Why can't running be like sex? Why can't I remember how good it felt last time? I think the reason is because, where running is concerned, I spend the first ten minutes thinking 'This *&@n' sucks!'

There is a fantastic rush that accompanies a good, long, sweaty workout. Unfortunately, it will take me at least two months of training to get to a place where I feel I'm doing more than working my way towards a heart attack.

I remember how running gave me more energy. I remember how once I became active, I wanted to *remain* active and was therefore a more productive father, husband and human being. But, man, at the end of the day, I'm just too pooped.

My daughter begins kindergarten in two weeks. As a result, it will be the first time in seven years both kids will be out of the house for 31 hours and 40 minutes each week.

I'll have no excuse.

Certainly not when I face that group of moms who gather outside the school brandishing Lululemon running gear and Bluetooth headphones linked to their MP3 players.

I have an MP3 player.

And shorts.

And shoes with a little, bright red Velcro tag with my home address and phone number on it so the medics know whom to call once they revive me. Some parents find the time; others don't.

Some parents make the time; others can't

How do you do it? *Do* you do it?

I know I should, especially now that I have the time. Of

course, we're redoing the entrance way this fall. I don't know how long that will take...but I can certainly arrange to work on it for 31 hours and 40 minutes a week.

CHAPTER 11

Phantom Symptoms – Myth or Fact?

The Boy Who Cried Wolf: Maybe he was really seeing them?

Why do we get itchy? There are medical reasons: allergies, sensitivities to certain fabrics, reactions to minor toxins released by insect bites such as mosquitoes, etc. Sometimes something is literally rubbing us the wrong way: a tag on a t-shirt, wool from a sweater, an in-law—all sorts of irritants. The real science behind a plain, unprovoked itch is not fully understood. Messages are sent to the brain, which interprets those messages in a certain way, to which the response is to tell your fingernails—or if you're a bear, a nearby tree—to take care of the problem. The cause can also be psychosomatic, which my ever-reliable 'Wiktionary' describes conveniently as pertaining to both the mind and the body. It is the same phenomenon that causes one to yawn in the presence of another who is yawning, or to cough or clear one's throat in the presence of someone who…you get the idea. A great place to witness this phenomenon is in a movie theatre. Do you ever notice that when one person feels the need to clear one's throat, the room becomes a sea of 'ahem's and 'hm-hm's? Even as I write this, I scratched myself at the beginning of the paragraph and cleared my throat during the last sentence. Do you ever watch a movie featuring swarms of bugs or a documentary on spiders and find yourself recoiling because you could *swear* you felt one crawling on your arm? Me, too.

That, dear readers, is a phantom symptom.

Now, here I am, an expectant father, who, for nine months, is living the most intimate moments of my life with someone who is experiencing regular bouts of nausea, headaches, back pain, leg cramps and a host of other symptoms born of pregnancy. Some of those feelings and those physical reactions are bound to rub off. The real skill is identifying and partitioning what is real from what is imagined; what requires treatment from what can be willed away; what should be kept personal and what should be shamelessly complained about to the pregnant person lying next to me on the couch. The wrong choice at the wrong moment can, in a worst-case scenario, deteriorate into a stressful argument with your pregnant spouse over a headache. It is an awkward situation when a husband is lying on the coach with his eyes closed trying to soothe the pain in his head, and his pregnant wife asks him to make her a cup of tea and fetch some Tylenol from the upstairs vanity. Advice to Dad: Don't answer "REALLY!? Can't you see I have a headache?"

In the best of cases, it *may* illicit sympathy from a woman whose abdomen is being distended farther every second by the human being nesting in her cervix. But that can be touch-and-go.

Dealing with your own discomfort during your wife's pregnancy can be tricky. But these scenarios are inevitable.

Sometimes, whether the trigger is psychosomatic or physical, your symptom won't present itself until your wife mentions hers. For instance:

Man and pregnant woman are lying on the couch. (There's a lot of lying on a couch in our house.) The woman lets out a groan. The man asks:

-"'You okay?"

-"Just a little nauseous," the pregnant woman answers.

Man acknowledges nausea with a soothing 'hmmm' and

perhaps a gentle rub of her back or her cheek, and asks if there is anything he can do. Then, perhaps, he gives her feet a little rub.

Moments later, the man begins to feel nauseous…truly nauseous.

A bizarre form of panic sets in. It is a mixture of excitement—the type a scientist must experience when he accidentally happens upon an illuminating result he didn't expect—and of fear that you may vomit on your nauseous, pregnant wife.

Phantom symptoms are not something men can discuss freely with their pregnant wives because, really, what pregnant, constantly nauseated woman wants to hear about her slim, suddenly nauseous husband? Nor are these symptoms something they can discuss with their male counterparts, for fear of being laughed off the basketball court:

-"Guys, I don't think I can keep coming to the pick-up games."

-"Why not?"

-"I've been suffering from my wife's morning sickness."

As much as women believe men have a sounding board in their male counterparts, the scope is somewhat limited. Everyone knows men—especially those men's own partners—well enough to be able to imagine the reaction from his cronies when he asks them: "Do you ever feel that your own symptoms of physical and emotional discomfort mirror those of your pregnant wife?" As much as I try to avoid profanity, the absolute, universal response would be: "F&?!, no."

There is another option for a man who needs to share his feelings in order to not only find answers but perhaps relieve the stress of the physical symptoms: Seek the advice of a mental health professional. One can only imagine the reaction a psychologist would have upon hearing—

-"Hi, my name is Kenny, and when my pregnant wife says 'I'm nauseated.' I, too, feel like throwing up."

The answer would most likely be:

-"Take a Gravol. Get over yourself. That'll be $250.00, please."

Or worse:

-"Maybe you need some time to yourself. Can you get out with your friends? Find an activity? A pick-up basketball game, maybe."

The dilemma is even more of a minefield when your wife is forced by a crushing migraine to take a trip to the emergency room, and suddenly, the hand-holding husband feels an intense headache coming on.

A little background on these pains-in-the-cranium from someone who, until a couple of years ago, wasn't giving them their due. I used to give someone who complained of migraines a sideways glance. I was a skeptic. It always seemed to me the migraine was merely a headache that was conveniently serious enough to allow people to get out of reporting to work for a day or two, while still allowing them to watch movies and eat junk food on the couch. 'I get headaches, too.' I thought. 'Take two aspirin and call us in the morning, right? Just like the rest of us.' Missing work or a dinner or a family gathering because of a headache? Please.

The real severity of a migraine was one of the many lessons I learned after being married to a brave woman; someone who was a steadfast non-complainer, a more-the-merrier sort. The *only* time I had ever seen her succumb to physical pain was because of a migraine.

Migraines are brutal, debilitating headaches that can cause not only dizziness, but more nausea and vomiting (oh, joy) than even the pregnancy itself, as well as temporarily blurred or reduced vision. Normally, there are some wonder drugs out there that can help such as nonsteroidal anti-inflammatory drugs (NSAIDs), triptans, ergots, anti-nausea medications, butalbital combinations and opiates.[6]

What's available to a pregnant woman? Tylenol.

What if, despite lying in a dark room and after taking Tylenol, you are still seeing a third head on your husband? It's time to seek hospital treatment.

Unfortunately for us, what should have been a relatively quick trip to the ER, turned into an all-night affair because of a group of jackasses.

At three in the afternoon, my wife felt it building. It began with a blurring of her peripheral vision. From experience, she knew this was stage one of the migraine to follow. Normally, she would pop a couple of Tylenol with codeine. But, alas, thanks to the lad within her belly, no codeine for her, just straight, plain old acetaminophen, then wait.

Two hours later the vision problem had indeed become a sledgehammer of a migraine. A telephone consult confirmed that if we (of course, in this case I mean the royal *we*) are to hope for any relief, *we* are going to have to present ourselves to the emergency room and receive an IV drip. The drip is safe

---

6   http://www.mayoclinic.com/health/migraine-headache/
DS00120/DSECTION=8

for pregnant women, and within a couple of hours it should alleviate the migraine. We were doubly assured that, generally, pregnant women are seen rather quickly, so our stay should not be extended to any unreasonable length.

No problem. I was only too happy to oblige. After all, I was in fine spirits and, as unbelievable as this sounds, I always saw a trip to the ER—in a supporting role—as a pleasurable outing. This may sound strange, but as long as I was the healthy person, and my reason for being there was not life-and-death (while a migraine is no picnic for the sufferer, she *would* come out of it alive), I quite enjoyed finding the nearest coffee station, grabbing the most recent of the old magazines off the chipped, melamine hospital table, holding my wife's hand with whichever of mine wasn't clamped onto a latte and letting time quietly slip by.

If you believe in God, the previous paragraph may be why He invented phantom symptoms: To give the guy with the latte a taste of what the person next to him is feeling. Not only to give him a taste of a migraine but also see to it that it would be best if Captain Coffee kept his discomfort to himself.

The pain hadn't hit me yet, but our night was far from over.

I checked us in with the bravado and sense of entitlement that every man feels when he is representing an infirm pregnant woman: *"WE ARE PREGNANT...WE ARE NOT WELL. WE MUST SEE A DOCTOR."*

We were sent to our little chairs to wait our turn.

We waited. And waited. And waited.

Finally, I had no choice but to ramp things up to Phase Two:

-"Excuse me," I repeated with an added edge to my voice,

"My wife is six months pregnant, suffering from a horrible migraine. We have been here two hours and have yet to be seen by *anyone*."

The receptionist's expression was so bland you would have thought I had just reminded her that after night follows day and then night again.

No kidding, pal. Get in line.

Been waiting? Take a look around, buddy.

It was true. The ER was swamped. An ambulance seemed to be rolling into the emergency bay every 10 minutes. From where I was sitting, I could not see the extent or types of injuries that were jumping the queue, just that there were many of them.

Finally, after my third or fourth complaint, I became a squeaky enough wheel to warrant being moved to a private waiting area.

The room was the size of a walk-in closet. A coldly functional exam table hugged one wall. Opposite the table were equipment cupboards and a sink. The remaining wall, opposite the door, supported an old, upright medical scale and a chair. My wife lay down on the table, eyes closed, her head resting on a hospital pillow manufactured by the same company that provides those small, polyester cushions to airlines. I covered her with a hospital blanket, compliments of a similar airline company. I was where I was supposed to be: seated next to her in the dark room, sipping cold coffee and being supportive if only by being as quiet as possible.

Two more hours passed.

Finally, a doctor stopped by. After he politely and gently asked the right questions, and we politely and quietly provided the answers, treatment was forthcoming. Intravenous medication would be administered. It was a small bag of liquid that would empty itself into my wife's bloodstream within about half-an-hour. Fifteen minutes after that, he would be by to check in. If the pain had not sufficiently subsided, the treatment could be safely repeated two more times. Then we would be sent home, headache or not.

I don't know if it was because of curiosity or frustration, but we asked what all the tumult was in the ER and why it had taken four hours to be seen.

The answer? Jackasses.

"Jackass" was, at the time, among the most popular reality shows on television. It had spawned an equally successful real-ity-based motion picture. It involved a troupe of young males who challenged themselves—and sometimes others—to test their limits of tolerance for physical discomfort. Some of the trials included eating glass, throwing themselves down stairs, eating more glass and allowing themselves to be kicked—and I mean NFL style—in the testicles.

Not only did this show live in the digital media, but it had also given birth to a traveling road show, with the participants performing feats of madness live onstage for a rabid audience.

As with most acts of pure insanity, imitation becomes a form of flattery. That night, the road show had performed at a local theater. After the show, the freaks and geeks in attendance had spilled out onto the downtown streets, possibly hoping to earn a spot in the next "Jackass" sequel. People were allowing their feet to be run over by cars, they had invited their friends to hit them over the heads with beer bottles and they juggled everything from knives to Molotov cocktails. Most daredevils found themselves in line at the emergency room—without a movie contract—just ahead of a pregnant woman suffering from a migraine, along with her healthy, obliging husband.

No one ever said that there was moral justice during triage.

The IV meds began draining themselves into my wife's arm as she lay with a towel covering her eyes, desperately trying to ignore the din of the triage area and the busy hospital hallway. I sat dutifully in my chair. My wife would every so often look in my direction and manage to utter words of comfort and encouragement to *me, the guy in the chair enjoying a coffee...!* She was a trooper.

That is about when it happened—about half-way thought the first IV drip.

I asked how she was feeling; was the medication helping at all? She said it was hard to tell; she didn't think so. She followed with similar questions of me. As I was replying 'fine' or something of the sort, I felt it: a headache.

The pain increased in the same fashion as Dr. Seuss described the Whos' singing in "How the Grinch Stole Christmas": It started in low, and it started to grow.

Eventually the back of my head felt as though it contained a small man whacking a tuning fork. The longer I sat and tried not to think about it, the more intense the pain grew.

I am a believer in the power of positive thinking being able to will away pain. A friend, who was trying to emphasize the existence of such a phenomenon, asked me if, by concentrating on a particular source of pain, I could make it more intense. I tried (I had strained my back moving some furniture), and sure enough, if I focused on the area, the pain became more intense. He, therefore, reasoned that if thought could intensify pain, it could also dull it or even make it disappear. This made sense to me, though I could never seem to fully put it into practice. Then again, I also believed that if I had a pain in my wrist, you could stomp on my toes and I'd forget all about it.

The first bag of IV meds was now empty. We waited in the dark for the doctor to return; I could tell my wife was doing no better. Her eyes were still closed and her furrowed brow betrayed the pain she was still feeling. I knew we weren't going home just yet.

The doctor poked his head back in, and with a soft-spoken tone to his voice that comes only with experience dealing with genuine pain, asked my wife if there was any improvement. She answered, almost guiltily, that there had been no real progress in the war against The Migraine. He told her not to worry; he'd be right back with another round of meds. He then looked my way with a smile, perhaps offering a little empathy from a married man and obliging caregiver.

"And, how are you?" he asked.

How was I, exactly? The truth is I had a pretty bad headache. It was due, no doubt, to fatigue, stress and a little dehydration. Anyone in a similar situation would have had a similar headache. But I had an advantage of being in a hospital ER; I was mere yards from a wealth of painkillers and only feet from a man with the power to write a prescription or at least find me a couple of Tylenol. The question was this: Do I tell the truth? Can I sit in a room next to a pregnant woman who is paralyzed by pain, with a needle in her arm, and have the temerity to say "I have a headache"? Do I seek relief or do I suck it up in the name of selfless support and lie?

"I'm fine." I answered.

I felt it was the right thing to say; the only thing to say. There are moments in life when the people around you who need your support and strength far outweigh your own immediate gratification. Black and white. Night and day. There are absolute truths in this world.

The doctor left to get more meds. It took two more rounds of treatment before my wife was well enough to stand and return home, after eight hours in the emergency room.

Those darn jackasses.

My pattern of phantom symptoms continued throughout the pregnancy, though under less extreme circumstances. There were times, as we wordlessly watched television in the evening, she would have a slight wave of nausea. After a few minutes, *I* would start to feel queasy. I would feel a cramp when she was crampy, felt hungry when she was hungry, and felt myself turned off by the sight of food after she claimed she had no appetite.

Why?

I would like to believe it was due to my sensitive, selfless nature; that I was so in tune and caring in the face of my wife's condition that every change, tick or wave triggered a similar reaction in me due to our strong psychological and spiritual connection.

Or maybe I am a big baby.

Maybe I did have a selfish, childish streak in me that was screaming for attention, and my subconscious was triggering these responses so I felt I had the right to complain. Was it all the physical equivalent of a foot-stomping five-year-old? I chose to think not. I credited a close relationship. But there was that part of me that looked forward to nine months from then, when I could start whining openly again.

ᐧ SELF-HELP TIP FOR THE iDAD ᐧ
Find an outlet: Run, Bike, Swim, Draw, Write, Sculpt.
It makes ignoring headaches easier.

CHAPTER 12

Jeeves, I'll Have an Espresso, or Husband Host Fatigue

Ilooove coffee. Coffee is my cigarette. Want to go shopping for bras? No problem, *if* I can stop first for a double-long espresso with a dash of hot milk and a pinch of sugar. A sale at Dorothy Perkins? Triple shot, large, skim, no-foam latte. Dessert and coffee? I don't have much of a sweet tooth, but if it's followed by a dark-roast, full-bodied brew with a little milk and sugar, I'll hang around for the mille-feuilles.

Before we go any further, here it is for the record: Espresso beans *do* contain more caffeine than regular beans, but since the water is infused more quickly through espresso grounds, and an espresso is (or at least *should* be) smaller than a regular cup of coffee, there is *less* caffeine in a brewed cup of espresso than in a regular cup of coffee. Although, when you order a triple-shot....

My wife and I cultivated our relationship with the help of the latte. If it weren't for 'going for coffee,' we may never have gotten around to talking with each other. Over the years, we've spent as much on coffee makers (Bodum French presses, stove-top espresso makers, percolators; another French press to replace the one that shattered, another stove-top model to replace the one that melted to the stove-top burner, etc.) as we have on retirement savings. The most I have ever paid for a few sips of Java was seven dollars for a single shot of Jamaica Mountain Blue coffee at a small shop around the corner. After seeing it listed on the menu, I ordered it, determined to cynically reject this expensive swill as a scam and fully expecting the product to be indiscernible from any other house blend available on the market.

I was, unfortunately, very wrong.

But I still can't justify forking out that kind of dough for coffee on a regular basis.

My point: As much as I love coffee—and as much as I love the ritual of brewing coffee and sitting down with a newspaper—as with a nine-month pregnancy, one can have too much of a good thing.

Our parents are all at least semi-retired. They are also all divorced. And with the exception of my father-in-law, they all live within an hour's drive. This is a mixed blessing because, while it will no doubt provide us with a wealth of baby-sitting in the future, it also means the week can fill up quickly with visits and phone calls. Remember, this baby is the first to be born on my side of the family and the first to come along in more than a decade on hers. This means the excitement and curiosity levels from the whole extended family tree are fairly high. This manifests itself with a minimum of a half-dozen phone calls and at least three home visits per week.

I understand how lucky we are. There are families separated by hundreds of miles, children who've lost their parents at an early age and other unfortunate situations that deprive parents-to-be, and eventually young grandchildren, of contact with their immediate families. This will not be the case for us. This child will have the love and attention of several generations for years to come.

BUT...

These frequent visits from individual camps can result in host-fatigue in an expectant father. This becomes especially prevalent during the first and third trimesters. These are the periods when the woman is generally most incapacitated. During the first trimester this is due to the ills that accompany morning sickness and other ailments brought on by the body's adjustment to pregnancy. During the third trimester it is the sheer size of the fetus that limits a mother's mobility and causes back pain, side pain and pelvic floor pain as well as general fatigue and fed-up-ness. By default, her condition necessitates the husband becoming more responsible for hosting and communication duties. These frequent family and family-in-law visits see the slow, steady transformation of a father-to-be into a part-time butler.

Welcoming people into my home generally brings me pleasure. I enjoy cooking and hosting and not having to drive home afterward. One of the real pleasures of a get-together is the sharing of lives and moments: listening to each others' stories, reveling in the happy details of a friend's life, or commiserating and supporting a friend in a time of trouble or despair. Mealtime is a wonderful opportunity for this type of bonding. The shared meal provides not only a topic of conversation but also a backdrop for the listener while soaking in the details. Your closest friends are always those who take an interest in you and your life. It is said, the most interesting person at a party is the person who makes you feel as though you are the most interesting person at a party.

It is when your role as host is diminished to butler that welcoming people into your home is no longer a welcoming prospect. Such became the pattern during my wife's pregnancy.

At first, the man is at least asked: 'How are you feeling?' or 'Are you excited?' or 'Have you told many people at work?' And we are included in the general conversations about the baby: 'Have you chosen a name?' or 'What color will you paint the room?' or 'Have you bought a crib?'

After said pleasantries, it is only polite for the man—who is, without question, in far better condition to host than a pregnant woman dealing with morning sickness—to offer some hors d'oeuvres and drinks, or coffee. So, that's what I would do.

-"Would anyone like something to eat or drink? Coffee, maybe?"

Generally someone would accept, if tentatively: "Only if you're having something."

Has any host ever responded to that with "Well as it turns out, I'm not having anything, so let's just talk."? Of course I'll have something. That's what one does when one offers food and drink to guests; one joins them. To do otherwise is slightly rude and more than a little weird.

But we all understand these rituals are all part of the host/ guest Olympics.

Off I would head to the kitchen to put together a low-maintenance snack plate: some crackers and cheese, some fruit and—since it is my parent or in-law visiting, therefore allowing for certain informalities—any leftovers that may still be short of their best-before dates (or not too far past them). The offer of coffee was also floated and generally accepted. We had recently received a new espresso machine, so the excitement of brewing a latte and hearing the sucking and frothing sounds of steaming milk was still fresh. I admit, I generally urged our guests to let me upgrade them from a pedestrian brew to something a little more sophisticated and Italian sounding. But the question "Would you like some coffee?" would soon become one of those questions to which I would not want the answer.

After a few weeks went by, a mathematical formula developed: $X = 1/Y$, where X represented the number of coffees served and Y represented the genuine interest shown by the server.

A directly inverse proportion.

In other words: With every coffee served, the father-to-be was taking less and less pride in making the perfect espresso and beginning to feel more and more like a simple butler.

There was a running joke between my wife and me. Every time in-laws or parents stopped by to lend us a hand or simply pay us a visit, I was relegated to coffee-and-snack duty in the kitchen, to be seen from that point on only through the convenient hole cut in the wall between the kitchen and living room. It was through that hole that I would serve coffee. I still remember the day our contractor/architect suggested that hole as a way of "opening up the space." Great, we thought, someone can be in the kitchen yet not be cut off from the conversation in the living room. Now I wanted to take that architect/contractor—who was not licensed in this country—and wall him up in that part of the kitchen like that guy did to his buddy in the wine cellar of Edgar Allan Poe's "The Cask of Amontillado." Burying my contractor would result in that hole being closed and also meting out the appropriate punishment for he who banished me to the espresso station.

She thought I was exaggerating my feelings of coffee-prisonership. I insisted I was not.

An experiment was in order.

166

One day her mother was on her way up the outside walk. I smiled at my wife, and said:

-"Watch this. Your mother will walk through the door, give me a passing 'Hello' on her way to give you a kiss (I used to get a peck on the cheek, as well, but that was prior to procuring the espresso maker) and in one way or another, send me to the kitchen."

My wife accepted the bet (although we never had time in these situations to decide on a prize for the winner or a punishment for the loser. This is one of the difficulties of betting against someone with whom you have a joint bank account).

In walked her mother—right past me to greet her daughter and ask her how she was feeling. The first words out of my mouth were routine with every visit:

-"Hi, how are you? Would you like a coffee?"

-"Sure! I'd love one! Thanks!"

-"Snack?"

-"Well, only if you were going to put something together for yourself."

One could argue, I prompted the service request by asking her if she would like a cup of coffee. True. But it's a Catch-22: The offering is part of the expected ritual. *Not* offering is rude. With no offer, when family members would finally be in their cars on the way home (months after they arrived, it seemed), they would lament—and correctly so—that despite their efforts to come and visit and maybe help with some chores around the house or even bring (yet another) baby gift, they weren't offered so much as a cup of coffee. Kenny really doesn't seem to help out much. I've read enough Dear Abby to know that if a snack was not at least offered, I would be 'he husband who's mean to his mother-in law.'

So I trotted, visit after visit, from the door, to the kitchen, to the living room with the snacks, to the kitchen for refills, to the living room, to the kitchen for clean-up, to the door for good-byes.

Thanks for dropping by. Now I have a headache. Great, phantom symptom!

Let's be clear. These menial chores are *still* more desirable than bouts of morning sickness or back pains and other spasms brought on by the weight of a seven-pound fetus, but the frustrations are still real.

Trying to find empathy in fellow men can prove fruitless. The unspoken secret is this: Men can be just as nasty where gossip is concerned as women.

There are three camps of men who complain about their wives:

Camp 1—The iDADs and iHUBBYs (Husbands with Emotional Intelligence): They love their wives. They live every moment with them, and as with any interpersonal relationship, there are some rough spots. When this camp comes together, it is not so much to share 'war stories' but rather to seek empathy from other people who also go through brief spats of frustration, which are expected when you share a home with someone. Phrases often spoken in this circle are "I still love her, but..." or "It's not something that happens often, but...."

Camp 2—The Silent Sufferers: Men who are internally experiencing emotions similar to those in Camp 1. However, they fear Camp 3 and, therefore, tend to err on the side of caution and choose to not share their frustrations at all with other men. The only anecdotes made public are those of an uplifting sort: Love the wife, love the kids. All is well. Roses are red and violets are blue." Pleasant, but unnatural.

Camp 3—The Boors: Unfortunately, this group still comprises a healthy chunk of the male population: those who have not outgrown adolescence and perhaps never will. They met their wives at an early age, found themselves uncontrollably physically attracted to them, which forced them into their best behavior, so they married them and became fathers. They did not foresee life after becoming a parent—much less life after several years of marriage—in any way changing from what it was as a 22-year-old college student. They somehow manage to seek each other out. They still live for televised sports and drinking nights with their buddies—to the exclusion of their family life. Everyone needs an outlet, but the Boor knows no limits. When you try to approach the Boor about domestic difficulties, the response is often as follows: "What do you care!? You have a job, too. You have a right to relax. I'd also like to be at home pregnant, lying on the couch all day. I'll be damned if after working all day, I'm gonna come home and start making coffee for my mother-in-law. You should go on strike, dude. By the way, are you in for the NFL triple-header on Sunday?"

Anyway. All that to say this: It is hard for the iDAD to find the right time, place and person in front of whom we can vent minor frustrations. I suppose we don't so much gossip, as much as we turn quickly to venting or to silence.

And try finding a sympathetic audience among exhausted pregnant ladies and excited mothers-in-law.

-"You're not the one who's about to put something the size of a snow blower out of a hole the size of an anthill."

Sometimes a father-to-be just wants to be part of the party.

Then again, we should be careful what we wish for because the parties will come, and when they do, there is no place to hide.

ᐧ SELF-HELP TIP FOR THE iDAD ᐧ

Speak up! Family visits are also a great time to sneak in a long, hot shower or a walk around the block. *Then*, make the coffee.

BACK FROM THE FUTURE
From Blog to Book

Inspired by the MenGetPregnantToo.com Post: The Relationship Bank: Is a Manicure Worth the NFL Conference Finals?
Published: December 6, 2011

The Relationship Bank begins with the ebb and flow of withdrawals and deposits from the moment a couple is on their first date. The balance in The Bank represents the amount of autonomous decision making and freedom each party has within the relationship.

Before kids are in the picture, an example might be like this: On the first date *he* drove, picked the restaurant, ordered the wine and paid the bill. In doing so, he deposited a certain amount into the relationship bank.

How much each party must deposit before expecting a return on the investment is entirely dependent on the couple—and often follows no rationale whatsoever. If the two of you follow more traditional dating and relationship guidelines, a couple of Olympic Games could go by before the other party cashes in.

Other methods of deposit are surprising your partner with flowers, giving massages, remembering she loves Leonard Cohen and surprising her with tickets while *not* offhandedly mentioning the outrageous cost of ticket prices nowadays.

The person who has made the largest deposits can eventually start making withdrawals. Last week you picked her up, brought her flowers, paid for supper and went to see a foreign film she's been drooling over (you also forgot your glasses, so reading two hours of subtitles made you lose your taste for popcorn and gave you a migraine). *This* week, you want to stay in, order pizza and watch the *Batman* Trilogy—again.

And so it goes.

Once kids are in the picture—especially after the first year—The Bank not only plays a more important role in the relationship; it becomes a near necessity.

Whether you are a parent working in an office and coming home to young children, or your job is to *stay* at home with young children, the lack of personal downtime can be overwhelming. The Bank allows each of you to remember you are still an adult who needs fulfillment and not just a parent fulfilling a child's needs.

An example from the blog:

My wife, last week, went for a facial at 2:30 p.m.—the hour one of us would be normally obliged to walk with our 4-year-old daughter to pick up our 7-year-old son at school, take care of homework and snack and start thinking about supper. No big deal for me; it was a nice enough day for a brisk walk and certainly more fun than the activity I was engaged in at the time—stripping wallpaper. But still, for this service, a small deposit was made (virtually and psychologically) into my account in our relationship bank.

As for my bank, it's pretty even; except for that trip to France my wife took when our son was 7 months old. That's a deposit that is still feeding off interest. And the spa facial? The NFL Conference Finals are coming up... an afternoon on the sofa with potato chips and the NFL? Mmmmmm.

During pregnancy, however, all bets are off. The changes taking place in woman's body can be so unpredictable that a father-to-be's attempt at planning 'selfish time' becomes near-

173

ly impossible. A couple of televised football games could be feasible. A round or two of golf should be manageable—much like football, it's no more than an eight-hour block. But, a week in France, a weekend in Vegas? Those are a little harder to justify, especially later into the pregnancy. A father-to-be is always conscious of those two infamous words: 'What if.'

What if something goes wrong? What if there's an emergency? The emergency needn't be of a medical nature; what if the basement floods, or the roof springs a leak, or that propane tank you should never have stored in the garage in the first place blows up?

Yes, any adult is fully capable of calling the insurance company, dealing with the adjuster or even turning off the water and soaking up the mess. However, playing Mike Holmes becomes far more challenging during the 7th month of gestation.

During pregnancy, consider The Bank closed—one nine-month-long bank holiday.

CHAPTER 13

Lessons From a Baby Shower, or One Million Ways to Say "Cute!"

· PET PEEVE OF THE iDAD ·

The men who don't show up at these functions
and the iDAD who can't leave.

Is it possible that while each sex is making long, overdue inroads into areas formerly dominated by the other—the most common being women full-time in the workplace and men as primary caregivers in the home—we have denied there are certain experiences, situations and emotions that are better suited, and quite simply preferred, by only one of the sexes?

Baby showers may be one of those occasions.

While every iDAD welcomes a ceremony celebrating the upcoming birth of his child, the shower—in its current format—is a definitively female activity.

Men know it and women know it. But like so many stages of the pregnancy and birthing process, there lacks an honest review and revision of cultural standards and expectations. Both men and women forsake honest admissions of their feelings in favor of points gained in the battle of the sexes. This battle has not diminished since the sexual revolution but has rather become more passive-aggressive and cloaked in its nature. The difficulty arises when, in these modern times, the progressive man suggests he may be better served spending the afternoon with friends outside the home rather than attending certain 'special' occasions: a baby shower, for instance. And the progressive woman may not realize—or chooses to not admit—that her husband may, in fact, be better served spending the afternoon with friends outside the home rather than squirming throughout a baby shower. In the 21st century, the baby shower has begun to swing from a unisex (women only, thank you), to a co-ed "Jackand Jill" format. Though the swing is gaining momentum, the pendulum is letting out squeaky complaints due to centuries of rust accumulation on the hinges.

Invitations to these showers are either sent solely to women, ignoring the husbands completely, or sent to the couple with much higher expectations placed on the woman's attendance than the man's.

Why? Because the baby shower is still seen as a celebration of another stage of *maternity* and not a stage during the transition into *parenting*.

An example of this is the level to which women versus men are expected to be involved in the actual planning of the event. In our case, the baby shower was kept a surprise from my wife, whereas I received a call basically asking me to plan the event. The call was from my wife's best friend and includedthese questions:

-"Who should we invite?"

-"What does *she* need?"

-"Can you call half the people on the list?"

-"What should *we* serve?"

It makes sense that a father-to-be, who is *not* carting 35 pounds of baby in his belly for nine months, be more active in the planning of an event than his pregnant wife. I am happy to have a nuts-and-bolts role to play in a shower to honor my baby. The disconnection occurs in the behavior that pretends the woman does not occupy a place of honor at the table relative to her hubby. The dynamic that would develop at *our* little celebration certainly supports the hypothesis that a man at a baby shower is like a ninth arm on an octopus; Yes, he *looks* like he belongs; yes, he serves a function, but sometimes he just seems he's getting in the way.

Traditionally, mothers-to-be are not involved in the planning of their own baby showers.

As part of a fair exchange, traditionally, fathers-to-be are not *present* for their wives' baby showers.

Yet, I was determined to meet role-reversal head-on.

I was the only one with such determination.

At each home I called, the conversation with the husband-half of the couple was the same:

-"Hey! I'm calling about the baby shower."

-"Cool, when is it?"

-"Two weeks from Sunday."

-"Cool! I'm sure Sue would love to go. I'll pass on the message. So, you up for a round of golf? Wanna hit a movie? Watcha wanna do?"

-"What do you mean? Now?"

-"No. The Sunday of the shower."

-"Well...I'm going to be at the shower."

-"WHAT? You got screwed, dude."

It occurred to me that the guest list suggested by my wife's friend didn't include *any* men. No husbands. No boyfriends. No fathers.

What was even more peculiar is that, where my attendance was concerned, the women had the same surprised reaction as the men. When I explained to them my mother-in-law would take my wife shopping the morning of the event while I remained at home welcoming guests and preparing for the surprise, even the women adopted an odd tone to their voices:

-"Oh, you'll be there...? Ummm, you know what? Good for you; most men go out for the afternoon."

I know. Thanks.

§

As guests arrived at the shower, I began to feel out of place, though I had trouble understanding why until much later.

I don't think there is any doubt that, within our biology, or nature, or spirit—whatever you want to call it—men and women have very different energies. Neither is necessarily more agreeable than the other, and, in the right mix, a wonderful balance is achieved between the two. Once the front door was closed and the headcount complete, there were twenty women, and me.

Any woman who denies there is a unique chemistry and atmosphere created when twenty women are in a room together is just plain lying. The same would be true were it a room full of men. The timbre of the room was different; there was an aura created that distinctly followed the predominantly female air in my living room and kitchen.

My wife was not home yet. I immediately changed gears and became restaurant owner, caterer, maitre d', coat-check person, Walmart greeter, furniture fetcher and butler. There was a buzz about when my wife would be expected home. How much was there to get ready? What final touches were needed to make the surprise perfect? Requests were made of me by the dozens: This goes in the freezer. This goes in the fridge. Hide this in the bedroom, and of course "Where's the coffee?"

Where's the coffee??? Never mind the coffee; where are your husbands?!

Once my wife was home, the party was in full swing. People began to take their seats, and the presents were lined up.

I headed to the kitchen to make another pot of coffee and to fetch the hors d'oeuvres and desserts. I was followed to the kitchen by a brigade invitees who had contributed snacks stored in my fridge. They were now offering their suggestions as to what kind of plate, bowl or glass would be best for showcasing their delectable contributions.

One rather yummy-looking pie sat in the back of the fridge in a springform pan. It occurred to me that although my male friends may be enjoying themselves in a movie theatre or sitting in their basements watching a football game in dirty boxer shorts, they're also missing out on what appeared to be a fabulous spread.

§

There are certain inventions for which I hope their inventors became millionaires. The springform pan is one of them. Pure genius. Anyone who has ever pulled something out of an oven and wrestled around the edges of the creation with a knife trying to free it from the pan without ending up with a slaughtered mess, owes a moment of thanks to the springform pan. The mechanism is brilliant in its simplicity. Place the base in the slot around the bottom of the interlocking band, flip the latch and voilà: a round cake pan. Now you simply bake your cake, pull it out of the oven, let it cool, flip the latch back and voilà: a perfectly round dessert with no sign of the desecration brought on by an impatient husband with a butter knife.

HOWEVER. Should one reach into one's refrigerator during a baby shower to retrieve a dessert generously donated by one of the guests, and should said dessert still be in the springform pan into which it was baked, one should be certain the latch on the pan is still in the locked position, lest the following take place:

My fingers, which were underneath the pan supporting its weight, accidentally popped the base out of the inter-*locking* band. The dessert went flying about four feet across the kitchen landing remarkably on its bottom, with the pan base still nestled underneath. The dessert itself was not solid to begin with but rather made with a yummy, moussy, jell-o-like consistency. The whole thing landed on the floor with a distinct *splat* and compacted downwards and outwards onto the floor in all directions.

There was then a reaction from my mother's friend who had baked the dessert and then transported it in the pan to the shower: "Kenny, I could kill you!"

At that moment, there were 20 women gathering over my shoulder hoping to catch a glimpse of the dessert catastrophe caused by the only male in the group. All of them had their own version of either a sarcastic cheer, advice on how to clean the mess or a joke about how men can't even get dessert right. Being the center of this kind of attention, coupled with the thought of my fellow dads waking up alone in their own basements in front of their TVs covered in Cheetos and drool, made me want to cry at my own baby shower. So what? Don't women love men who show emotion?

At this point, any guest who may have been unaware of the kitchen calamity was now jogging to our small galley kitchen to see what it was that had finally led to Kenny's demise.

What's worse than trying to clean up two pounds of yummy, mousy, jell-o-like substance off your uneven, industrial slate kitchen floor? Doing so with 20 female baby-shower guests glowering over you suggesting (or not) how the clean-up should proceed. I would have warmly welcomed a male guest at that point, if only for a sympathetic look and to hold the mop.

Fortunately, there were enough other desserts (and plenty of coffee) to go around.

We eventually took our seats, ready for the ritualistic opening of the gifts. Of course, now the comments won't stop: "Kenny, don't drop anything!" "Kenny, maybe you should just watch!" "Kenny, don't touch anything breakable!"

Nothing brings people together like collective ragging on an outsider.

It would have been nice to hear: "Kenny, why don't you go see a movie with my husband?"

§

Stocking up on supplies for your first child can be costly, both emotionally and financially. Although most things are not necessary—almost any piece of furniture can be used as a change table—other things you cannot do without: feeding paraphernalia, a healthy stock of diapers and wipes, bottles, etc. We are very lucky to have a generous circle of friends who drowned us with gifts that day.

That being said, when gifts are purchased for adults—for example, for an adult birthday party—the reaction will vary appropriately for each gift. For a piece of clothing: "This will look great." For a new Blu-Ray collection: "I can't wait to watch this," For a gift certificate: "I love this store."

However at a baby shower, though the gifts are just as appreciated—and even more necessary—they all pretty much demand the same reaction, especially where baby clothing is concerned: "CUTE!"

Alone among a group of 20 women, I was fascinated and impressed with how all of them were able to conjure the same level of excitement and appreciation for the 14th blue onesie with a bear on the chest as they had for the first. Yes, yes, I know you can't *not* show appreciation; after all it is a gift. This person went to the store, took the time to buy this item and wrap it and brought it to your home. But, at that moment, if I had turned the word 'cute' into a drinking game, I never would have made it past the first 10 gifts. I would later comment to my wife that someone should invent a little pop gun, which every time you pulled the trigger it would yell 'CUTE!' with great enthusiasm. Perhaps on some score sheet, having disdain for the repeated mention of the word 'cute' would show up as 'insensitive' in a box of male faults, but I felt distinctly awkward mustering the same level of excitement as my female guests. I think other *male* guests would have felt similarly—had there been any.

Is this because my upbringing made me incapable of emotionally giving in to the moment? Is it because our society teaches men to be cynical when faced with a pile of baby clothes? Is it biological? Is the male brain simply not designed to appreciate the beauty of 14 blue onesies? Are the women faking it?

I don't know the correct answer; I just know how I felt. My thoughts kept straying back to the springform pan explosion. My inner monologue kept reassuring me it wasn't my fault. After all, I didn't *open* the latch, which means it was never closed tightly enough to begin with, right?

During moments of daydreaming during the gift opening, I began to people-watch. My eyes scanned the circle of friends. The shower was also a window into the relationships and reactions women had toward each other: The experienced mothers reminisced; the single women either checked their watches or did their best not to look melancholy—or at the very least distracted—and women of my mother's generation compared notes about the successes of their adult children with all the subtlety and competitiveness of racecar drivers.

Maybe I wasn't the only one dealing with infant product overkill. It was very believable, even likely, that the single women would return home and talk to their single friends about the hysteria that surrounds the unveiling of 14 baby tops. They probably feel hopeful about the day when they, too, will be the focus of a baby shower, or some may feel sadness at the thought that they may never have children. Others will feel joy and relief with their decision to not become mothers.

Me? I was back at the espresso-maker brewing some decaf, waiting to thank the guests, show them out the door and begin cleaning up, unless anyone wanted to stay after the party for a refill of our famous bottomless cup of coffee.

⁃ **SELF-HELP TIP FOR THE iDAD** ⁃

If the husbands decline the invitation to your shower, threaten them. Tell them to get over here or the friendship is over. Also, beware the springform pan.

CHAPTER 14

No Epidural for Stress

· PET PEEVE OF THE iDAD ·

When, along with a small suitcase, my emotional baggage
makes a trip to the hospital.

Even for iDADs, the final two weeks of a pregnancy are very emotional. The feelings run the gamut and can change from moment to moment: boredom, fatigue, impatience, nervousness, fear and anxiety. I imagine the feelings are similar for pregnant women.

Aside from the extreme physical discomfort and fatigue my wife was experiencing—thanks to the small human nestled in her abdomen—both our psyches were, by and large, being put through similar drills. When is the baby coming? Was that pain a labor pain or just a pain? Is the bag packed? Did we forget anything? Why won't our parents accept 'we'll let you know when the baby comes' as a truthful answer and stop calling several times a day?

As the husband, I found it challenging to provide enough support and care for my wife, to be sure she wasn't lacking for either while at the same time trying not to drive her crazy by asking too often: "How are you? Are you OK? Tired? Can I get you anything?"

After a while, I think she was hoping to give birth to an alien that would jump out and get me off her back. Wanna bet the alien would ask for a coffee?

The alien never came. So we paced, lay around and talked about the baby until we didn't want to talk about the baby anymore.

Then, on November 9th at 11 p.m., the pains started to come. At first, they were intense but infrequent. On the phone, the hospital told us they were too infrequent to justify coming in; we would just end up waiting around. (Personally, if I'm in intense, albeit infrequent pain, I'd rather wait around within a few yards of a medical professional than next to my husband who works as a TV producer, but I understood that a couch in our living room is probably better than a waiting room or a gurney in a hallway.) A couple of hours later, the pains became more intense, bordering on unbearable, and they also came more frequently. On the phone again, the hospital said the contractions were still too infrequent to justify coming in.

If I had to euphemistically translate my thought at that moment, it would be "I disagree with that. Let's go!" Otherwise known as "F&^* that s&*@. Let's go."

I enjoyed being at the hospital in the middle of the night for the same reason I enjoyed arriving at the airport too early for an early morning flight or enjoyed working at the office on a weekend: It was quiet. These hospitals, which are normally homes to noise—both human and non—bathed in fluorescent light and fed on a diet of urgency, accomplishment and failure during their peak hours, lie mostly silent at 2 a.m. A hospital at night can be more peaceful than a library. The lights are dim, the hallways empty. Patients are, by and large, asleep, and the minimal staff murmur amongst themselves at the nurse's station. Unfortunately, the cafeteria is also closed, so the only coffee available is from a machine, which I swear was a gas pump in a former life.

Any peaceful feeling I was experiencing was somewhat diminished by my pregnant wife's grimaces of pain and the fact I was moments away from being responsible for another human being for the rest of my life.

We approached the nurse's station of the maternity ward. I

explained to staff that my wife was nine months pregnant and was having painful contractions at five-minute intervals. Though they had told us that we should wait at home, her unbearable pain overrode any chance of our obeying that suggestion. The nurse smiled warmly while I spoke and guided us to a small exam room.

There were 88,400 births in Quebec last year distributed over 66 maternity hospitals. That means, given equal distribution, this hospital serviced 1,339 of those births. If this nurse works full-time, that is to say five eight-hour shifts a week, she has been on the job for more than 250 births so far this year (including a two-week absence for vacation). Here I was, the 251st father to be explaining to her for the 251st time that we were at home, my wife was in pain and we had called the hospital... blah, blah, blah. To her credit, any monotony she felt, she didn't show.

The exam 'room' consisted of two beds, foot-to-foot, with enough space between them for a curtain and enough room beside them for a chair, a fetal and maternal heart monitor and a couple of extra inches ensuring the door didn't hit the occupant of the chair in the head.

My wife lay down. She was fitted with the appropriate monitoring equipment and nestled her feet under the pile of our coats at the end of the bed. My position was what would become my home for the next four days—a pleather hospital chair next to my wife.

It is at this stage that a father-to-be's role undergoes an interesting transformation. At home, during the day-to-day operations of a forty-week pregnancy, a father fancies himself a person of importance. Even if we are not physically pregnant, we draw energy from the experience. At work we become the guy who's going to be a daddy. At home we try to be the pillar of support: the chef, the masseur, the caretaker. Now, in the hospital, we become absolutely powerless. Should there be any change in my wife's condition, I would have but one option: go and tell someone about the change in my wife's condition. Outside that responsibility, I would have to go into Moneypenny mode: Call our closest friends, call our parents and try to convince them (the parents, anyway) they don't need to be here yet—the doctors say it could be a while. During that 'while,' I should try to keep my wife as comfortable as possible—both emotionally and physically.

I was actually having a great time. I felt exactly the way I do in the early morning hours at the airport; I was excited for the journey ahead. I had done all I could do as far as preparation was concerned, and tomorrow at this time I was going to be in a wonderful place. Little did I know, this hospital stay was going to be closer to a near-death experience than it would be to a vacation.

§

I continued to do what I could:

-"How are you feeling?" I asked.

-"Not bad. Not great but not bad," she answered.

-"A lot of pain?"

-"During the contractions, yes. But, other than that, I'm just tired."

I told my wife I was going to take a walk around the joint—maybe see about getting a beverage out of one of those things that used to double as a gas pump. Would she like anything?

-"A magazine, please."

Cool. Off I went.

Amazingly, I did find a 24-hour newsstand that sold various publications as well as non-perishable snacks and cold drinks—no coffee. The man working the night shift at the hospital news-stand directed me to the machine down the hall. My wife is always interested in news and current events, so I quickly grabbed a couple of titles and headed back to the room.

In unusual situations, people behave unusually. My wife was certainly not herself—she was in tremendous pain, and though she is never one to complain, the strain was understand-ably showing on her face and in her body language—her eyes were closed, she was taking deep breaths, and yet still she said she was feeling "not bad."

The husband's behavior, however, during these stressful situations, was much freer to manifest itself in unusual ways. After all, I was not in mortal pain, bound to a bed, attached to wires displaying not only signs of my stress but that of the human being stuffed inside me.

I handed her the chosen magazine.

She said: "What's this?"

-"What's what?" I answered.

- "This is all they had?"

As I took the magazine from her to verify its contents, it occurred to me that prior to purchasing it, I never really looked at it, I had just taken care not to buy something that had the image of Betty and Veronica, or Scooby-Doo, or Jane Roe and Henry Wade on the cover.

I immediately noticed why she was objecting. I had bought a political publication that focused on prison torture and the subsequent mental breakdown suffered by those being tortured.

Oops.

-"Here, try this one." I said, honestly not really knowing if my second choice was any better, rather just having faith that by not focusing on physical torture, the second magazine was, by definition, an improvement.

-"It's ok; don't worry about it," she said. "I'm just going to close my eyes, anyway."

I sat back in my pleather chair, took the magazine for myself and learned more than I needed to learn about prison torture.

§

For four hours we waited in that room. The contractions were coming more steadily, and with each one my wife's face registered the pain. During that time, another woman and her husband were shown to the bed opposite to ours. She, too, was subsequently strapped with monitor wires. He tumbled into his pleather; he, being the 252nd person this year to explain his 'unique' situation to the duty nurse. We heard their conversation:

-"How are you feeling?" he asked.

-"Not bad. Not great, but not bad," she answered.

-"A lot of pain?"

-"During the contractions, yes. But, other than that, I'm just tired."

I considered offering her a magazine but reconsidered.

I took solace in realizing the universal ritual of the moment. Even though, for my wife and me, this was a first-time experience—both unique and terrifying, the birth of a first child is something completely foreign to the parents-to-be; it is a feeling never to be repeated. Yet three feet away from us was another couple, similar to us in age, related to us by their worry and fear, experiencing something so identical to us in almost every way.

There have been nearly four billion births since 1960. I cannot think of another event that presents such a dichotomy: All parents have experienced birth, yet everyone is able to tell a story of how the experience is unique for each of them.

The maternity nurse looked at the readout on the tapes being steadily expelled by the monitors—a sort of electronic paper regurgitation.

There was now a birthing room available for us. We walked—very slowly—down the hall, the flight towards parenthood beginning its second stage.

§

This room was big; it was a private room designed to be both waiting room and delivery room. The bed was in the center surrounded by all the necessary equipment for the birthing team. The bed was almost like a creature. It had a removable foot with stirrups tucked underneath, arms for IV drips, storage spaces for medical equipment, plenty of room on either side for a large team of physicians and nurses and whoever else may be needed in an emergency. Even for me there was an upgrade; in the corner, pushed up against a wall next to a window, was a chair: pleather, with a footrest, though this one fully reclined to transform into a small pleather bed.

We'd moved into our new home. My wife was helped onto the bed. I was the able porter, fetching our bags and settling into my pleather throne.

-"Need anything?"

-"No," she answered.

Men, this is a key to avoiding having to do chores: if you mess up the first errand really badly, they don't send you out on another one. The prison torture magazine may have just saved me a trip to some gloomy part of the hospital on some other mission.

They offered my wife an epidural.

What follows is not a verbatim recounting of the conversation, but I have tried to capture the spirit of the moment.

-"Do you need something for the pain?" said the nurse.

-"DID NEAL ARMSTRONG NEED PROTECTION FROM THE VACCUM OF SPACE?!" my wife answered.

-"I'll be right back," replied the nurse.

§

Have I mentioned, I've never been good with needles?

But this isn't about me My wife needs drugs.

Before they inserted the epidural, they wanted to start an IV in a vein on the back of her hand. I reported for duty next to my wife and held her free hand. The needle was huge. I told myself not to be bothered by it; this is about her, not me. I certainly was not about to tell my wife 'I know you're in excruciating pain, but I can't hold your hand and support you. I think I'm going to pass out. Deal with it, please. I'll be in my pleather chair.' So I held her hand and tried to look away. But, like a rubber-necker passing a car accident, I couldn't help but peak. All I could do was take some deep breaths and hope to not pull her off the bed with me should I lose consciousness. Worst case scenario, I thought I would just flop on top of her. This room was so big I was too far from my fine, pleathered friend for him to be of any help.

Once the intravenous was successfully started in her arm, it was time for the epidural. I felt a mixture of sympathy for my wife—who was leaning forward off the side of the bed onto my shoulder, being told not to move while a needle was being inserted into her spine—and an immense sense of helplessness. It seemed unfair that I was not being put through some form of procedure myself, just to even the odds.

The drugs were a miracle. She was given control of a pump, through which she could regulate, within reason, the amount of painkiller being administered into her bloodstream. Her thumbs had never gotten such a workout. The pain was subsiding to the point where she was now relaxed and reclined in her automatically adjustable bed, waiting for the human being in her belly to squeeze through a hole the size of a tangerine. She slept. I, however, had nothing to do now but watch the readouts and listen to the subtle beeps of the monitors. One displayed the rate of my wife's heartbeat, another was for the baby's heartbeat, and a third measured the intensity and frequency of the contractions. I had with me books and music and headphones and a radio, but I was fixated by the readouts on these machines. I had no idea the adventure I was about to embark upon. First though, there was a situation in the waiting room to deal with.

§

My parents are divorced. Much like the juggling that took place when they were first informed of the pregnancy, juggling their relationship during the hours prior to the birth of their first grandchild was tricky. The pattern of controlling and balancing the flow of information to each of them was something I'd gotten used to. Firstly, it required two phone calls and two conversations to inform them of any news, big or small: change of jobs, change of address, being home with the flu, how am I feeling after being home with the flu for three days? How are you feeling two weeks after the flu subsides? Who's this girl you're seeing? When's the wedding?

You get the idea.

Secondly, and most importantly, having them in the same room made me tense. I felt responsible for ensuring that they each had time with me and that they were enjoying themselves at whatever event we may all be attending (especially if I'm the host). I understood that, as an adult, it was not my responsibility to see to their happiness, but where our parents are concerned, do we ever stop being children?

They have now each received two phone calls. The first

was when we were headed to the hospital. The second was when my wife was moved to the birthing room. In both instances, they were told what we were told by the doctors: She has not yet begun to dilate, so we're still hours from giving birth.

They heeded the advice to stay home after the first phone call. After the second, though, they couldn't hold out any longer. I believe there was a certain competitiveness motivating their early arrival at the hospital waiting room. One would not want to arrive hours after the other; this would make one seem less interested—a less loving parent. So as a result, I now had my divorced parents sitting in the waiting room, where they may well be waiting side-by-side for the next several hours. This should not be my problem; I have a wife and fetus to be with. But childhood guilt and a sense of responsibility is making me feel very tense about the situation.

Fortunately, they are not forced to sit shoulder-to-shoulder. My closest friend, who received the same two phone calls, also chose to err on the side of caution and be in the waiting room, just in case. Not only has he arrived early, but he has taken up a position between my parents. He's the human embodiment of the United Nations.

Shortly thereafter, my mother-in-law arrives. She is the antithesis of my parents. Whereas my family will sit quietly, passively waiting for updates, my mom-in-law has all the quiet passivity of livestock in Pamplona.

She was, at one point during the pregnancy, pushing to be in the delivery room. My wife was considering allowing her to join in the proceedings, but I fought against it. This is our baby—mine and my wife's. This story would be ours to tell. I felt my mother-in-law, having given birth to three children herself, already had her mental and emotional birthing experience. I felt it wrong that, sometime in the future over Christmas dinner, while I was recounting the story of my son's birth, Mom-in-law could jump in with "That's not how I remember it." It wasn't an easy argument to win. Although the baby was 50 percent me, an extra 20 percent of convincing was needed to avoid my in-law sharing in 33.3 percent of the experience. Mom-in-law, if we ever take the kid to Italy—and can afford the extra ticket—you're in. But for now, no, you cannot be in the delivery room.

But I now felt an uncomfortable dynamic developing in the waiting room: My mother-in-law's daughter is in a birthing room with a needle in her back, another needle in her arm and monitors attached to her belly. A couple of hours ago she was in tremendous pain and would still be if not for medication. This was mom-in-law's only daughter. The same way we may never stop being children around our parents, they never stop being parents around their children. Besides having a biological attachment to the patient in the birthing room, mom-in-law is a cheerful, energetic person and not a worrier by nature. Allowing her in for visits in the birthing room was not only the right thing to do, it alleviated a little bit of the responsibility I felt, since it was difficult to be alert and present for every minute of what was becoming a long, slow labor process. Plus, now that my wife was in a drug-facilitated slumber and in the company of her mother, I could grab my buddy from his peace-keeping mission and go raid the gas-pump/coffee machine.

My parents, though, were definitely exuding an air of people being left out of the developing situation. They watched

Mom-in-law move in and out of the birthing room, and now I was watching them watch her move in and out of the birthing room. I did not want to exclude them, nor did I want to bring them in together and watch them stand side-by-side ignoring each other. And I did not feel like turning one trip by a parent into the birthing room into three individual trips. I tried my best to let them deal with the situation and tried my best to—just this once—not let their being bothered bother me. They became easier to ignore as the medical situation in our birthing room began to deteriorate.

§

It was now past noon on November 10th. We had been in the hospital for 10 hours. Although the contractions were coming more quickly, my wife was still not dilated enough for the baby to pass through the birth canal.

After my welcome walk around the hospital and a visit to the swill machine, I was ready to resume my post in the pleather recliner. I kicked Mom-in-law back to the waiting room and let my eyes alternate between my sleeping wife and the monitors next to her bed.

I began to notice a trend: each time the contraction monitor spiked, the fetal heart monitor would slow. I watched as one machine went beep-beep-beep, the other would slow proportionally: beep—beep—beep.

Next time the staff checked on her, I mentioned the trend in my best 'I'm no doctor, but this seems odd' voice. They confirmed the baby's heartbeat was slowing with each contraction, but reassured me it was not to a dangerous level. They said it was best to let nature take its course before administering any more drugs. The next step would be to induce labor, which would hopefully encourage dilation. But let's wait a couple of hours.

This meant two more hours of updates to the forces in the waiting room, where the party now included my sister, and two more hours of sitting in the pleather chair watching my baby's heartbeat slow as my wife's abdominal muscles squeezed him.

§

Suppertime on the 10th. Hospital arrival time plus 16 hours.

The doctors were now in the corner of our room, conferring in hushed tones about how best to proceed. The contractions were now frequent enough, but my wife's cervix was still not sufficiently dilated. Meanwhile, the baby's heartbeat continued to slow dramatically with each contraction. Although my wife was still in no real discomfort—thanks to the drugs—my anxiety level was rising as I strained to hear the impolite, private conversation in the corner.

I understand why doctors didn't want me in on the conversation. The same hierarchical rules apply around the world, in all situations. In summer camp, the counselors meet without the campers and the program directors meet without the counselors. In schools, teachers meet without the students and the board of directors meets without the teachers. In government, the cabinet meets without, well, all of us. The reason being that, by-and-large, the public is prone to hysteria and irrationality. Although these qualities are by no means absent as one ascends the societal pyramid, they are hopefully less likely.

I was not included in the hushed conversation in the corner because a) I had absolutely no medical expertise to bring to the table, and b) they didn't need a hysterical father interrupting the flow of decision making with emotional outbursts. That being said, I fancied myself a logical, intelligent fellow, who I thought capable of listening quietly to a conversation concerning the life of my wife and unborn child. I knew that of myself, but they didn't know that of me, so I was confined to the pleather. There was also the possibility that my opinion of myself was biased and incorrect, and that I was prone to shrew-like outbursts, though I'd never seen it happen.

The doctors broke the huddle and explained they should not allow the labor pattern to continue much longer. They were going to break her water *manually* with the hope that that would further induce dilation and accelerate the birth.

I answered: "OK."

From my pleather throne, I watched the doctor adjust the foot of the bed and prepare for the procedure. I would have gotten closer, except that this was a teaching hospital, and any spot that would normally be reserved for the comforting husband was taken up by doctors in various stages of an incomplete education and a couple of nurses who not only assisted the doctor performing the procedure but also ensured that those there to learn didn't get in the way. By way of sliding something resembling a knitting needle through her cervix, the amniotic sack in my wife's uterus was pierced, and the fluid that had been a soothing hot tub for my unborn son for the past 40 weeks drained into a tray.

Now, we wait, said the doctor.

I answered: "OK."

Another trip into the waiting room, another update, another trip into the birthing room for Mom-in-law, another impatient shift in their chairs from my silent parents.

Two more hours passed. The same trend continued: more contractions, a slower heartbeat, no further dilation. The doctors were back. Another conference in the corner of the room. I began to wonder why they couldn't meet in the hallway. Then, at least, I wouldn't have been as aware that there existed a situation requiring a conference with a staff of medical experts.

The doctor explained that breaking my wife's water has not only *not* helped, but the lack of fluid around the fetus may now eventually pose a danger. What they were going to perform now was a relatively new procedure whereby the amniotic fluid removed hours earlier is reinserted. Not to worry, he explained, this was not a dangerous procedure. The doctor assisting him proudly pointed out that the team leader is one of the only doctors in North America who has performed this procedure.

Should this not work, I'm told, the last resort is a caesarean section.

I answer: "OK."

This time I didn't make a trip to the waiting room. I'd been watching my wife undergo intense contractions for nearly 20 hours and been watching my son's heartbeat drop to what I perceived to be dangerously low rhythms for the past six. I was also getting the feeling that the doctor's calm demeanor was masking what was becoming a more and more critical situation.

Like a chef with a turkey baster, the doctor re-infused the

fluid.

Now, he said, we wait another short while.

I was beginning to feel fairly done waiting. I asked why we don't automatically proceed with the c-section. Surgery is always the last resort, I'm told.

Frankly, with the way I was feeling at that point, if that hospital room was a vacation spot, I would have named it 'The Last Resort.' I felt like screaming, 'Will somebody please take this baby out!?'

Instead I answer: "OK."

§

Midnight, the first minute of November 11th— Veteran's Day. Twenty-two hours since our arrival at the duty nurses station. Two-hundred-forty-two babies have been born in this province since we checked in. We still didn't have ours.

The fluid removal and re-insertion had done nothing. My wife's cervix had not dilated to more than six centimeters; no full-term baby can fit through a hole only six centimeters wide, certainly not any full-term baby with my wife's genes: Genetically, her family has large heads.

The doctor said they will follow through on the decision to perform a caesarean section. He told us not to worry; we should be brought into the operating room within an hour or two and everything should be fine. They were going to be back to check on us in a little while to fill us in on what is required.

-"OK."

This time I did make a trip to the waiting room and kept

it short. There were rumblings of questions from the gallery, but I didn't have any more information to give them. Also, my anxiety level was too high to allow me to stand there and issue a State of the Nation address.

I return to my pleather chair to wait.

About an hour after the doctor had told us there was no hurry, a small team of medical staffers burst into the room and insisted we head into the operating room *now*. *Right now*.

I pictured some chief of something receiving a briefing of the situation in our room and yelling at the staff for letting it go on this long. Imagining that scenario somehow gave validity to my own feelings. It was also likely that, given the state of medicine in this province, the operating room had just become available and we had to grab it before the friend of a friend of the chief of staff came in for a wart removal.

While they wheeled my wife and her bed down the hall toward the operating room, a nurse looked over her shoulder and issued orders to me:

-"Grab your personal belongings and bring them all into the recovery room across the hall. Don't leave anything behind. Take off any jewelry you're wearing and leave them in your bag in the recovery room. When you've done that, head to the end of the hallway, grab a set of scrubs and a mask, put them on and wait there. Don't move. Someone will come and get you."

I tried to be as understanding and calm as I could. Not only could I not think of any questions to ask, but the tone of her voice, and the pace at which they were moving my wife down the hall, clearly told me there was no time for questions. Minutes counted.

I obeyed the instructions and waited in a small plastic chair facing a wall of scrubs on shelves just outside a huge set of double doors that hid two operating rooms. I was cold and nervous. I don't know if the chills were due to the temperature in the hallway, due to my fatigue, or my nerves or a combination of the three. I waited for nearly 20 minutes. The longer I waited, the more I expected someone to apologize for forgetting I was out here and for forgetting to tell me the birth went fine and mother and baby were resting comfortably in the recovery room; your mother-in-law is with them.

A darker side of me was expecting to be informed of a crisis in the operating room, and that due to complications, things were not going well; it's best for you to wait out here.

Eventually, the nurse brought me through two sets of double doors and into the operating room. It was two in the morning. Outside the hospital, most people in the city were asleep; the hospital had the same peaceful quietness about it as it had 24 hours earlier when we first checked in. The operating room, however, had the bustle and activity of an airport during rush hour. The lighting blared, and a medical team was moving quickly about. There were quick, controlled conversations ,procedural in nature and professional in tone. An anesthetist sat next to a wall of machinery traced with graphs, lights and tubes. In the middle of it all was my wife, draped in sterile sheets. One sheet was clipped vertically two feet towards the ceiling across her chest, preventing her from watching the procedure.

For me, there was a momentary shock at the change in atmosphere. For the past full day, I had been sitting in plastic chairs, in dark hallways and dimly lit rooms while waiting for something to happen. This felt as though I had been woken from my bed and tossed onto a highway at high noon.

I was directed to a stool near my wife's right ear. She was woozy from medication but aware enough to send a little smile and hello my way. I was so glad to be there with her. All I could do was hold her hand, which seemed grossly insufficient, but I knew, at that moment, that's what she needed most.

§

They began the procedure. I was simultaneously curious and reticent to catch a glimpse of what was on the other side of the curtain. I knew peeking over the sheet at the wrong time would result in my wife's only human support system needing his own medical team to treat him as he lay on the floor. At the same time, I had a strange thought that if I *didn't* look over to see what was going on, I would somehow be sending the message I wasn't interested in the goings-on. Yes, I over-think everything.

Not wanting to be totally disassociated from the moment, I stood from my stool prepared to witness my first operation.

The anesthetist gently put his hand on my shoulder and said: "Stay seated please, sir."

Bless that man for taking the decision out of my hands. I was given no choice; I wasn't allowed to look at the blood. Where was this anesthetist that day when I was watching that educational video in college? Everyone should travel with their own anesthetist.

Whatever information I lacked due to my sequestration from the actual operation was being compensated for by developments and sensations on my side of the curtain.

As part of the side effects of the medications my wife was given during the operation, she developed a severe tremor. Her whole upper body was shaking as though she was in a field in the middle of winter. She was also cold and was developing a severe headache. The anesthetist gently asked her how she was doing and said he was making modifications to her medications to try and keep her as comfortable as possible. He told her not to hesitate to let him know if things didn't improve in the next minute or so. He was kind and attentive. Although she was probably his 200th patient this year, we were treated as his first. I was doing all I could to reassure her, which wasn't much. Her arms were strapped to the bed at near 90 degree angles from her body, ensuring she didn't move in such a way as to disconnect the intravenous lines. I held her hand, stroked her head and asked how she was feeling. Occasionally, my concentration drifted toward the action at the other end of the table.

Even though caesarean sections are considered major surgery, and incisions are being made around someone as delicate as a not-yet-newborn baby, the procedure is anything but delicate. Though I couldn't see what was going on, I could feel it. They were making an incision in a human body through which they would remove a small life form, though it felt more like a mechanic replacing a carburetor. My wife's body was jostled left and right with each tug and stretch. Though I could only see the doctor's top half, he appeared to be leaning over and reaching and pushing as though he was trying to pull Santa Claus out of a chimney. On and on they went: push, pull, left, right, put your hand here, give me that, there it is.

And finally...done.

From behind the curtain whooshed a nurse holding a baby. Still no sound from the baby, though.

Sometimes Hollywood movies take things too far, creating moments of suspense that are implausible—heroes rush in at the nick of time to save the day, or a baby is delivered but doesn't cry for the first few seconds just so the audience is forced to wonder whether the baby survived. I hate that kind of manipulation in movies. But those moments exist in movies for two reasons: First, audiences want escapism and drama and this adds to the film-going experience, and second, sometimes these scenarios really *do* happen in real life.

Like now.

For a moment or two I watched the nurse and doctor examine my silent son. Of course, I imagined the worst. I watched the last 24 hours unfold slowly with nothing but moments of suspense, a violent surgical procedure and dropping heart rates. It was almost inevitable that there be some casualty—either permanent or temporary—to either my wife or my son. I was convinced I would be going home with only one of them, though I didn't know which.

§

I was desperate to ask questions: Is everything OK? Why isn't he crying? Why the hushed tone among the medical staff? But I knew my questions would be anticipated, and demanding answers would only distract from the work being done to the small boy on the small table. My questions would also not change the outcome of whatever was to be. So I waited.

Only a minute went by, but as we've all experienced, during times of stress and anticipation, one minute seemed to take forever.

Then he cried.

-"Is he OK?" I allowed myself to ask.

There was no immediate answer, but seconds later while handing me a small bundle wrapped in a cotton blanket, the nurse answered:

-"He's fine. Congratulations."

I held him up slightly, trying to let my wife see his face. She was still tied down, I was still not allowed to stand, certainly not with a baby.

There we were, in an operating room, my wife with a hole in her belly and tubes in her arms and I holding our son. We're parents.

My stress level dropped like water from a broken dam. I was emotionally drained, relaxed and coddling my newborn while smiling at my spouse.

Now that my level of tension had dropped, I was able to stare at and stroke my baby boy, while listening to the procedure still going on on the other side of the curtain. I heard:

-"OK, we'll do 1, 2, 3, 4; then 5, 6, 7, 8....

I realized they were discussing where to put the staples that would hold together the various levels of my wife's innards. They were literally stapling her back together like an art project. She was feeling nothing. There was a hole in her belly; a team of people were stapling her shut, and she was feeling nothing. Suddenly any headaches, or nausea, or hosting fatigue I wrestled with during the previous nine months seemed laughingly insignificant.

§

Once my wife was put back together, they said they would bring her to the recovery room; I should meet them there.

Now, not only did I feel I was ready to face the gallery in the waiting room, I couldn't wait to see my friend and my family.

I pushed through the double doors to the waiting room. Voilà! I said. She's fine, he's fine, (and I'm fine). My buddy was making a video recording of my arrival in the waiting room like I was a groom walking down the aisle. There were hugs all around, kisses all around, congratulations all around. Everyone was asking to see mom and baby. Who goes first? Who cares? Let the recovery begin.

ˆ SELF-HELP TIP FOR THE iDAD ˆ
Waiting room politics have no room on your list of responsibilities. That's what double doors—and friends—are for.

CHAPTER 15

12 Steps to Recovery; 6 Floors to the Men's Shower

˙ PET PEEVE OF THE iDAD ˙

Father's attendance is preferred, but not necessary.

We spent a short time in the recovery room, one just wide enough for three beds—again separated by curtains—and enough clearance at the foot of the bed for a counter of supplies and a couple of visitors. Fortunately, or not, we had the room to ourselves. When I say 'ourselves' I refer to my wife, myself, our new son, my mother-in-law, my parents, my friend and my sister. It was a happy place. My wife, newly stitched, was being kept warm by a warming blanket—a sort of soft membrane into which warm air was being pumped from what looked like a leaf-blower. The baby, after being passed around, lay on his mother and breastfed for the first time.

We are not born knowing how to walk, or talk or support our heads, but we are born with the skills required to breathe and eat—perhaps this does something to explain the North American sedentary lifestyle; we spend a lot of time doing what comes most naturally, sitting and eating.

I felt tremendous joy, but after a short while, I also felt the need to be alone with my wife and the new member of our immediate family. I knew there were obligations to share the moment with the people in the room; they were thrilled for me and my wife, and it was the first baby born to my generation, on my side of the family. Despite this, I felt overwhelmed by the moment, and after the adrenaline had done its work, the fatigue of the event began to take over; it had been 26 hours since we first walked into the hospital. Also, I felt selfish, an emotion I wrestle with from time to time. It had been a long day, and I had spend most of it either being a messenger or worrying about the health of my wife and our unborn baby, while also trying to be a calm layman trusting in the words of doctors and nurses who were constantly conferring in the corner of our birthing room. I was ready now for some 'us' time. I wanted to spend some time with my wife, who had finally made it through a very trying ordeal, and my new son with whom I had yet to share a quiet moment. I had spent nine months getting to know him through the walls of my wife's abdomen, and now a small room-load of invited guests were accompanying us on our first steps together in the recovery room.

My sister and my friend were the first to leave; your peers are always the first to recognize when you're looking shifty and tired and need your space. The three remaining adults lingered. My wife seemed thankful for their presence, especially that of her mother—another example of how children never stop being children. I, however, was again feeling the anxiety of the moment. With only the parents remaining, and my mother-in-law by my wife's side, I was left talking to my parents. I, perhaps selfishly, wanted the room cleared. Is it right to feel this way? After all they, too, had been anticipating this moment for 40 weeks (nearly 33 years and 40 weeks), and were probably feeling as excited about the evening as I was. They had also spent 12 hours in the waiting room, and of course, for them, where else was there to be right now? Only bowling alleys are open at 2:30 a.m. and neither of my parents bowl. Still, I felt what I felt. Right or wrong, I wanted to exhale and relax my shoulders, but for some reason couldn't make that happen in present company.

Fortunately, the nursing staff—having dealt with similar situations more than 250 times this year—had their fingers on the pulse of the room. The time came to kick everyone out, and move my wife, the baby and me up to our room on the maternity ward. Party over.

§

Each medical professional we met throughout the pregnancy—from the technicians performing the first ultrasound to the doctors in the birthing room to the nurses in recovery—congratulated my wife and me on making me part of the process. I received kudos for my dedication, for taking the time off work to come to appointments, for being inquisitive, and generally for my love and support of the pregnancy and birthing process. This hospital often espoused the father being an integral part of the entire pregnancy and birthing process. It is your baby, too, they would say. We want the men to feel as necessary to the process as the women are, they would add. Now, we all know that men are not as *necessary* to the process; women around the world are managing well—and in some cases *choosing* to go through the whole procedure, including a lifetime of after-birth parenting—alone. However true or possible that may be, this hospital, and the staff we encountered, treated me like royalty for a) being there and b) being involved and willing to 'get my hands dirty' (while, for instance, remaining seated on my little stool in the operating room). The staff was conveying, in every way possible, that we were fulfilling the ideal scenario: husband and wife, equal partners in the raising of a child, from conception to adulthood and beyond. The physical building itself, however, was not necessarily in compliance with hospital philosophy.

§

First opened in 1893, the architect did not design the maternity ward wearing his 'Don't Forget the Fathers" T-shirt. Yes, we had a private room, the same way London, England, manages to have plenty of private hotel rooms. How do they do it? Maximizing the available space—each room being the size of a womb. Our room measured about 10 feet by 8 feet. This included an adjustable bed for my newly stitched wife, a bedside table, and a small bathroom. (Can we stop calling rooms without a bath 'bathrooms'? Again, the English have it right: it was a 'Water Closet'—the WC.) We also had a 'crib' for the baby (really a tray on wheels with glass sides nine inches high), all our personal belongings, and in the corner, a chair for the father. Orange pleather. We were to remain in the hospital for four days.

Of course, fathers are encouraged to stay with their wives and babies for the duration of their hospital stay; why would I want to be anywhere else? I've waited for this moment for 40 weeks. My entire life and 40 weeks. I've watched my wife and child go through what I perceived to be near death experiences. However naive and hysterical that may be, it was *my* perceived reality, and here they were by my side, alive and well and needing my support. *Even if* I was the kind of father (and you know you're out there) who *didn't* want to be here in this recovery room, how could I possibly feel right sleeping in our cozy bed at home, leaving my wife alone in this dark tiny room, unable to walk to the WC due to recent surgery, tending to a newborn baby alone for the first time in her life? By golly I was moving in! Even if it meant bonding with—and sticking to—another pleathered friend.

The chair, fortunately, was designed with a touch of Amish genius. Its wood frame and plastic 'pillows' could be reclined and rearranged to make a bed. The bed, when fully extended, measured about 5 feet long by 22 inches wide. I am 6 feet tall and about 20 inches wide. Also, although the 'bed' allowed its occupant to be fully reclined, my feet dangled well off the end. The whole contraption, when converted, had only 2 inches of ground clearance. The arms of the chair then became bedrails alongside my lower ribs and hips, making it difficult to change position and impossible to distance my arms from my body.

Look, I know the score. I'm not the one squeezing something the size of a watermelon out a hole the size of a grape. I get it. But (there's always a 'but' when men are uncomfortable) the scenario hardly supports the philosophy: 'In this room we welcome two new happy parents.' I would have been crazy to complain at the time; that's what writing a book is for.

The first night, the nurses offered to keep our baby in the nursery. "It's a one-night-only offer," they said. They would rather you kept your baby with you and began breast-feeding immediately, but they understand what the mother has been through and are offering to let you get one decent night's rest; it may be the only one you will have for months. We debated, even agonized slightly, but I convinced my wife to take them up on the offer. We'll have all the time in the world, I said. You've been awake, and either going through terrible labor or major surgery, for more than 30 hours; let your body rest. Our son was wheeled across the hall to the nursery and slept with pint-size roommates for the first night of his life.

§

I tried to settle into the pleather, but it was not going well. I was cold, uncomfortable and crowded. Plus, every time I changed position, my legs made a *peeeel-swwak* sound as they unglued from the vinyl. Unable to sleep, I crossed the hall to go visit The Boy.

As much as people make statements hinting that a newborn may look like one parent or the other, the only way I could identify my son was by scanning tags taped onto the cribs in the nursery. Had I been led to the wrong baby, I probably would have fawned and teared up just the same. Wrapped in blankets, with caps pulled down to their eyebrows, they all look very similar, especially to a parent who has only been a parent for four hours. Anyone who wonders why humans' skin pigmentation varies from culture to culture should visit a hospital nursery. The variation doesn't exist due to geophysical conditions, melanin or Darwinian lineage. It exists to help new fathers immediately recognize which babies are *not* theirs.

I greeted the nurse with an exhausted, affable smile that said, 'Hi, I'm Kenny, I'm a new dad. You won't believe what *I've* been through.' She greeted me with a polite nod and a "May I see your wristband, please?"

I was just one dad of 88,000 babies born in this province every year; we don't need war stories, just an I.D. bracelet.

What a surreal experience. I was, for all intents and purposes, making my first trip to my son's bedroom. How many times in the future would I make a similar trip to comfort him from nightmares, to change his wet sheets, to check on his fever, to pull the blanket up to his shoulders?

Here it was: Day 1. What business did I have, making myself responsible for someone else for the rest of my life? Yet, here we were. He was already dependent on me: Don't drop me; keep me warm; make sure I'm fed; keep me clean. The list would only get longer as the decades passed.

§

The second night, Baby was staying with Mom and Dad. By the second afternoon, I was ready for a scrub-down. I had not showered in three days. I did not want Baby to identify his father by some noxious, poisonous body odor. I put on my slippers, rummaged through our suitcase and rolled my shampoo and soap in a clean towel. I had packed for an extended stay; you never know. I walked the length of the hall, passed a door with the emblem that adorns the doors of women's bathrooms everywhere: a black figure with a round head, straight legs, straight arms and a triangle for a body. I headed in the other direction. Near the other end of the hall was another women's bathroom. This door was partly ajar. (When is a door not a door? When it's a jar!) I peeked in and was looking at a single room with a toilet and a shower stall. I assumed that, even though this was labeled a woman's shower, surely they wouldn't mind if a supportive husband—and new father recently recovering after witnessing (from his stool) an emergency caesarean section—used the facilities.

-"I'm sorry sir," a nurse said from down the hall, "those showers are reserved for the new mothers on the ward."

-"And where do the new fathers shower?"

-"Ninth floor, sir."

Six floors up.

OK. I understand.

After all, when you've squeezed something the size of a carry-on out of a hole the size of a ping pong ball, you don't want to limp down the hall only to find the shower occupied by an able-bodied dad enjoying his exfoliant. And, you know what? I'd been sitting around for days now; I was feeling a little muscle stiffness. I took the stairs to the ninth floor. It did me some good.

§

The ninth floor is a ghost town. It is abandoned, waiting desperately to star in the next Wes Craven film. There are few lights on in the hallway; the rooms are completely dark. I am feeling distinctly alone and a little creeped out.

When I was 11 years old, I stayed up to watch a midnight showing of *The Amityville Horror* on television. During a commercial break, I went upstairs alone to my room to change into my pajamas. ("You can stay up to watch as long as you're in your PJs before it's over. Then right to bed." Mother's instructions.) As I pulled my pajama bottoms on, my older brother kicked my door opened as hard as he could and screamed at the top of his lungs. I've never been so terrified.

Alone on the ninth floor of this hospital—built in 1893—a couple of butterflies in my belly reminded me of my idiot brother and The Night I Watched *The Amityville Horror*.

Finally, I happened by a door upon which is the universal sign for a men's bathroom: a black figure with a round head, straight arms, straight legs and straight body. I pushed the door open and discovered a corpse. OK, so I didn't really discover a corpse, but nearly as bad: Only cold water seems to run out of both taps. I assumed the last time this was used was in 1893, so I wait. And wait. No hot water. Surely, there was something I was not understanding. Or, at the very least, there were other showers around there somewhere (probably in the underground parking garage—mostly empty this time of night). I descended to the eighth floor to enquire further about the availability of a warm shower, which is available to men.

-"No, sir. This is the Women's Pavilion. Men's showers are on the ninth floor for reasons of privacy."

-"But there's no hot water on the ninth floor."

-"Oh, that could be; they're doing some construction up there."

Burying bodies, no doubt.

I pushed further: "Where are there other men's showers?"

-"Two pavilions over."

Did I mention this particular hospital is built into the side of a mountain? Two pavilions over means three different elevators and a couple of serious climbs. I'll deal with the cold water.

There's a wonderfully realistic scene in the movie *The Recruit* in which Colin Farrell, being recruited into the FBI, is thrown into a cold shower as a form of torture. His reaction is spectacular! He really sells you on the idea he's being tortured. How did he do it? The actor demanded they actually throw him into a real cold shower. Why simulate it when you can recreate the real thing and elicit an actual reaction of someone being tortured? Exactly. So went the thoughts in my head as I enjoyed the cold shower on the ninth floor of healthcare's answer to the Bates Motel.

I survived. After all, I'm not the one who squeezed something the size of a snare drum out of a hole the size of a kiwi. It's only a cold shower, not major surgery.

§

Back in our room, The Boy moved in for his first full night with Mom and Dad. As the lights went out, we alternated between my son nestling and feeding with my wife, him sleeping in his 'crib' and the little Jelly Bean all swaddled up and lying down with Dad on the fine pleathered bed.

When does a man hardly move? When he is forced into the clutches of a pleather couch-turned-cot. When does a man not even twitch? When he is forced into the clutches of a pleather couch-turned-cot and then handed his newborn son. I handled the overnight diaper changes as quietly as possible. I think my nervous heavy breathing was louder than his crying, and I think I used more wipes to remove the flop sweat from my brow than I did to clean the meconium from his bottom. The nurse, though, thought I was ready for my next challenge.

He was a healthy baby, though he had lost slightly more weight than the staff would have liked. Therefore, we were to supplement the breast milk with formula. I was excited by this idea, since it would enable me to participate in the feeding process. I imagined the bonding that would take place between my son and me as I reclined on my orange throne, nestled him in the crook of my arm and gave him a bottle. The nurses, however, had another idea. Perhaps they were taking revenge after learning I'd disturbed the staff five floors up while complaining about the shower six floors up. There would be no bottle for my son and me to bond over. Instead, there would be a little plastic cup. The reason they didn't want us using a bottle was, for a baby, going from an artificial nipple to a real one and back so soon after birth would confuse him. I was going to defend the bottle, explaining that any son of mine, born already knowing how to eat, is also born with an innate understanding of the differences between a latex nipple and a real one. And, as long as dinner was being served, he wouldn't be too fussy. But, who's asking me? I didn't want to be forced into another cold shower.

To feed him from the cup, I had to prop the guy on my lap, support his little chin with my sweaty hand (time for another shower) and tip the formula into his mouth $1/1,000,000^{th}$ of a teaspoon at a time. The challenge to doing this in the middle of the night was to be quiet enough to allow my wife a chance to sleep; after all, this was a big advantage for her to my being there. Whenever my son woke, I tried to be as quiet as possible, to get to the crying baby quickly, to swaddle him properly, to reset the pleather throne to its upright position, to pour the tablespoon of formula into the cup and balance both cup and baby as I walked across our 8-by-10 room that was littered with our personal belongings.

Once the feeding was done, I reversed the procedure to get The Boy back to his crib. I would then gingerly return the chair to its reclined position and hope to get some sleep. That was when I would hear The Sound: The *previous* meal had just arrived in The Boy's diaper. This was one of the first of several baby functions that I learned was normal but *must* have been designed purely as a practical joke aimed at parents: Newborns often pee and poo while—or just after—being fed. This period also coincides with the minutes following the application of a fresh diaper. Great.

§

Our third day in the hospital was when I came to yet another realization of what my wife had gone through. The nurse came to our room to change the bandages covering the incision from the c-section. Due to the lack of little 'queasy dad' stools in the room—as well as there being no one in the maternity ward knowing me well enough to suggest I don't watch—I stood at the end of the bed while the gauze was changed. There it was. An incision seven inches long, just above the pubic line. It was at this spot that a doctor had taken a scalpel and cut through my wife's skin, muscle, uterus and gestational sac and created a hole through which he pulled our son into the world. Unbelievable. I really needed a cold shower.

§

One of the advantages of the caesarean section—the risks of major surgery not withstanding—is that mothers are required to stay in the hospital for four days after the procedure. We, as first-time parents, saw this as a chance to get a few days of much needed neonatal education. Several-times-a-day visits by nurses gave us access to an encyclopedia of answers to all our questions: meconium, breast-feeding, diaper changing, bathing, dry skin, hair loss, umbilical cords and belly buttons. While I wouldn't suggest anyone undergo major surgery unless it is absolutely necessary, I also can imagine how much more nervous I would have been had I just been sent home cold turkey with a little guy about half the size of a cold turkey. There is nothing in anyone's life that requires more responsibility than caring for a child, yet you usually have about 24 hours after giving birth to get in your last-minute questions. Other than that, you are politely directed to seek help from the "New Mother" section at the bookstore, or as in "Who Wants to be a Millionaire?", you can phone a friend. Of course, you can make an appointment with your pediatrician, but you can't really bother a doctor with the day-to-day, small-fry questions about your Small Fry. Of course, there's the Internet, but with so many different opinions and so much information, you must have the patience to research, weigh and evaluate what everyone else has to say— not easily done for a sleep-deprived, nervous parent. Frankly, there is better phone support available for customers after they purchase a big-screen TV than there is easily accessible support for a new parent.

§

Last day. Time to go home and begin a new life as a three-some. Of course, there was the matter of removing a row of staples from my wife's belly.

The medical world is highly specialized and sterile, and for many of us laypeople, it is perceived as almost a magical world of healing. It's remarkable to notice that the equipment they use, while much cleaner, is not so far removed in design from what one would find in a garage or tool box. A stapler puts the staples in, and a pair of scissors and long tweezers take the staples out. Such care is taken to keep everything sterile; a sterile sheet covers the staples and sterile scissors are used to cut the staples that are then placed on a second sterile sheet. This sterile procedure is being performed in our room, on a woman who spent the last 96 hours next to a tiny, newborn meconium machine and a nervous sweaty husband sticking to a not-so-sterile pleather chair. It was like watching those people behind the fast food counters wearing those 'sterile' rubber gloves. Yes, they use the gloves to handle your food, but they also use them to touch the cash, the toaster, their utensils and their clothes. Really, all those gloves do is keep the employees hands clean from all the dirt falling onto your submarine sandwich.

Final check is done on the mother and the baby by nurses, gynecologists, general surgeons and pediatricians. Questions are asked about the home environment.

-"Do you have many stairs to walk at home?"

-"We live three floors up, but our condo is all on one level," my wife answers.

-"Will you have help getting the baby and your belongings

upstairs?"

I was standing right next to the interrogator, coat in hand. Apparently, my special power of invisibility was out of control, again.

-"My husband is with me."

-"Will you have help during your first little while at home?"

I was *still* standing right next to the interrogator, coat in hand. AHEM! HELLO!

-"My husband is taking five weeks off work."

-"Oh, that's nice. So, you have a support system waiting for you?"

HEELLOOOO???

My wife was more polite than I was about to be.

-"Yes, I'll be fine. We have lots of family. And my husband is very involved."

-"Good. Did you bring a car seat?"

I'm so involved, I think I'll involve myself in leaving the room and schlepping to get the car seat.

§

Here we were: my wife, the nurse, the baby and I, all gathered around the car seat, which I had placed on the bed. He was stuffed into his little snowsuit—which was four sizes too big (it was a gift; we were told he'd eventually grow into it)—and the nurse observed while I wrapped my first-ever, five-point harness around my first newborn baby. She couldn't let us leave unless she saw the baby properly secured—hospital policy. Of course, if I drove home like Mario Andretti, that was out of her hands.

Boy, was he squirmy. I instantly developed flop-sweat. I wasn't crazy about being observed. I wasn't crazy about breaking part of the baby with a five-point harness. I clicked all the buckles into place.

-"Tighter," said the nurse.

I pulled on the straps.

-"Tighter. You should only be able to get one finger between the strap and the baby."

Yeah? Which finger would that be? Wanna give me some space?

More sweat.

-"Don't worry, you won't hurt the baby. He's been curled up in a fetal position for nine months, so he won't mind the car seat."

Hmm. I never thought of it that way. That made sense to me. Of course. But while he may not mind the snug car seat, if he's been curled up in a womb for nine months, the fact that it's minus 5 degrees outside will come as no great joy to him. Welcome to life on the outside, son.

We finally got him strapped in and my brow wiped dry with the sleeve of my winter coat.

My father had offered to help us move home; after all, we had the baby, gifts, flowers and our suitcase. I refused. I wanted to walk into my home as a threesome. As much as it took three trips to the car to pack us up, I didn't want to share the moment with anyone other than my wife and son. I didn't want to make coffee for guests when we got home; I didn't want any suggestions from family members during our first moments together. I wanted a peaceful, quiet, pleasurable intensity that I felt would only come with being alongside the only other person experiencing these feelings—my wife.

So, we drove, unpursued, out of the parking lot.

As much as talking on a cell phone or texting may be a distraction behind the wheel, *nothing* is more distracting than having your first newborn in the back seat. I never stopped looking in the rearview mirror at his little face. Is he happy? Is he warm enough? Is he tied in properly? Is he really mine?

I've also never driven so cautiously. I could have been a driving instructor for Moses. Here's how to take 10 years to drive 10 miles: Creeping along, signal two blocks ahead of time, hands on the wheel at 10 o'clock and 2 o'clock. It was navigational perfection ad nauseum.

But at last we were home.

§

As we got settled into our house, one of the first things I noticed was the phone message waiting for us, the little light on the receiver going blink-blink-blink. I assumed it would be messages from the friends and family members who had not been to visit us at the hospital. I was surprised the messages were not from friends or even distant relatives but from the very same parents who had been with us off and on for the last four days. The same ones who showed so much concern for my wife's well-being during the last nine months (How is she?).

Their messages were by and large of the same theme:

-"Congratulations, you two. Your world is really about to change."

And their last line was always directed at my wife:
-"Let us know if she needs any help."

Epilogue

And THAT Was Just the Beginning

I supposed we do it to ourselves, we men. Too many of us are forced to rush back to work. Dare I say a number of new fathers *look forward* to getting back to work. I've watched my peers complain at dinner parties about how they don't go near a dirty diaper with a 10-foot-pole. How, after a week of work, Sunday afternoon is reserved for alone time—watching football and eating Kraft dinner. Mothers and children are told they can go visit the in-laws. For too many men, spending time with their newborns is limited to holding, cooing and bouncing, never the messy stuff: the cooking and cleaning and laundry and bathing. Is it time we use the designations 'Motherhood' and 'Fatherhood' less and start using 'Parenthood' more? Each parent will always have a unique style and place in the home, but taking care of a child is all-day, all-the-time, non-stop and forever. This is nothing new, but maybe the time has come to realize that parenting is, as much as is possible, 50/50. Even when one parent works outside the home, once work has ended for the day, the child is still half yours. Not only half yours but half *you.* There should be time in a relationship set aside for the couple, as well as for each parent individually, and that should be negotiated between the couple. But the outright refusal of certain childcare duties is an ancient concept. It's time for everyone to come to loving terms with meconium. Embrace the dirty diaper. Wallow in the spit-up. Wanting a child means wanting parenthood. A baby isn't a coin collection. Coin collections do not poop. They also will never hug you back.

Every baby has a biological father. Every father impacts the life of his child, whether he stays at home or works overtime, whether he is a fantastic husband and caring father or leaves the family at the first sign of trouble. Half of all the biological parents on the planet are men. Yet, for whatever reason, we are much slower to gather as a group and discuss the fine points of parenting. We don't get 'the guys' together on a regular basis to talk about our child's development or our own sleeplessness or stress. We don't share with our fellow fathers those moments of apprehension that may make us want to scream or cry. Many of us just stumble to the movie theater, constantly talking about how our wives are tired and how good it is to get out for a night. Many of us roll our eyes when our wives want us to read-up a little bit or when we feel our pregnant wives are too emotional.

We stand side-by-side, like a giant six-pack, 6-foot-tall bottles holding in all those same emotions and worries. How much easier would it be if we let ourselves be more emotion-ally elastic with each other? How much closer would the rela-tionship be between men and women—and between husbands and wives—if we learned to see that there may be more of the opposite sex in each of us than we first thought? The first step might be for us all to admit that while pregnancy is physically exhausting, becoming a parent is truly terrifying.

The End

Acknowledgements

At this moment, my children are 9 and 6 years old. This gives you some idea as to my level of self-doubt and constant procrastination throughout the process of finally releasing this book. It also means that, for nearly a decade, my closest friends and confidants have heard me say—in one form or another— "My book's almost done!"

Without a baby, there would be no book. Without my wife, there would be no baby and no book. Without her, I would be a man living in the two-room apartment I called home when we first met. I would be living there with a couple of cats (which I would no doubt keep replacing as nature did away with the old ones), staring out that window at an apartment block across the alley from mine. There, would live more men, with more cats.

Dale, I love you. I not only love you for the reasons that are mentioned in so many song lyrics and holiday cards, but I also loved when you patiently read and praised what I'd written. I loved when you cocked your head to the side and suggested changes. I loved when you became exasperated and said: "So, stop talking about it v

Letting your friends proofread and offer suggestions can be terrifying. Thank you, Rob G. for not only pushing and guiding and designing but mostly for laying the groundwork to the first 39 years of my life in order that I may be living this result. Bea, your unbridled enthusiasm about this book uplifted and encouraged me every time you offered it. Tracey and Rob B., you're proof that one doesn't require a lot of friends, as long as a person has the right ones.

In the online world, I have met no one as selfless and helpful as Lexie Lane. I met her, and a welcoming community of mothers, through her site: www.Voiceboks.com. They cheered every post I wrote. Lexie, you've made a career of putting other bloggers' needs before your own. In today's 'smash-and-grab' Internet age, you are a true gem.

Who would have thought I would have been touched by a group of four hundred or so digital friends? To the Dad Bloggers Facebook group (www.facebook.com/Dadbloggers), thank you for sharing your lows and successes and your skills and ideas, and thank you for all your selfless encouragement for those of us who need it most. Please visit their page for wonderful examples of talented male writers (who also happen to be dads).

Lynn Messina is proof that being generous with your time as well as with your experience can not only help the rookie author on the other end of the email but also create a lasting impression that will absolutely be paid forward.

Finally, Christine. You were a necessary floatation device and guide for a guy drowning in digital details. Thank you.

About The Author

Kenny Bodanis is the author of *MenGetPregnantToo.com*. The site's articles and interviews focus on the trend of shifting gender roles in parental duties and involvement, as well as such topics as bullying, stress, and other challenges facing both children and parents.

His blog was named by *Reader`s Digest Canada* as one of the top parenting blogs in the country—the only dad on the list. It has also received accolades in the U.S. and the U.K.

Kenny's column, "Questions Parents Ask," appears weekly at *LifeWorks.com.* He was part of a trio of bloggers at the site who won the Marcom Platinum Award for their writing.

He is also the regular parenting contributor for Montreal's *Breakfast Television.*

He lives in Montreal with his wife and two children. This is his first book.